Pedagogies of Widening Participation in Medical Settings

Addressing the fact that under-representation has been a concern for medical educators, medical councils, and the government for some time, this book presents the first evidence-based monograph for pedagogies that can be applied to all aspects of widening participation, tackling chronic under-representation in medical settings.

Discussing implications that have international ramifications for the field, the chapters showcase a variety of case studies, research, and evaluations that draw on experiences and insights from a wide range of current practitioners, exploring topics such as outreach, access, selection, retention, and progression. From widening participation leads and officers to national representative bodies and students from medical schools nationwide, the book sets out perspectives, guidelines, and research that can be applied throughout the medical student life cycle. Novel in approach and timely in content, this edited collection coincides with the drive to increase social mobility and the proportion of medical students from educationally and socially disadvantaged backgrounds, directly tackling the class system and elitism present in the medical professions.

This book will be of great benefit to scholars, researchers, and postgraduate students in the fields of medical education, multicultural education, and higher education, as well as those researching the idea of widening participation in the medical field and diversity in the professions more specifically.

Louise Alldridge is Associate Professor of Biomedical Sciences, Peninsula Medical School, University of Plymouth, UK. She is currently Widening Participation and Programme Lead for BMBS with Foundation Year, Peninsula Medical School.

Contemporary Pedagogies of Medical and Health Professions' Education

Series editors: Paul Crampton and John Tredinnick-Rowe

This novel series will focus on innovation and best practice in relation to curriculum design and teaching methodologies within the environments of medical schools, ultimately aiming to promote innovation in medical education. Books in the series offer cutting-edge examples of pedagogical techniques and practises through case studies and rigorous scholarship, and reflect subjects that medical schools are adapting in order to drive innovation such as the increasing role of patient-centred medicine or the expanding use of technology in medical curricula.

Themes identified in the series have international relevance given the similarities around educating medical students and their interaction with other clinical professions, and showcase novel research methodologies and frameworks to aid teaching and learning and preparedness of the next generation of clinical professionals.

Books in the series include

Pedagogies of Biomedical Science

A Holistic Approach to Integrating Pedagogy across the Curriculum
Edited by Donna Johnson

Pedagogies of Widening Participation in Medical Settings

Addressing Under-representation through Partnership and Professionalism
Edited by Louise Alldridge

For more information about the series, please visit: Contemporary Pedagogies of Medical and Health Professions' Education – Book Series – Routledge & CRC Press

Pedagogies of Widening Participation in Medical Settings

Addressing Under-representation through Partnership and Professionalism

Edited by Louise Alldridge

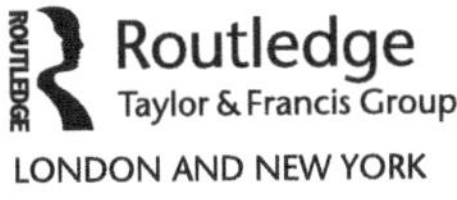

Routledge
Taylor & Francis Group

LONDON AND NEW YORK

First published 2025
by Routledge
4 Park Square, Milton Park, Abingdon, Oxon OX14 4RN

and by Routledge
605 Third Avenue, New York, NY 10158

Routledge is an imprint of the Taylor & Francis Group, an informa business

British Library Cataloguing-in-Publication Data
A catalogue record for this book is available from the British Library

ISBN: 978-1-032-49868-3 (hbk)
ISBN: 978-1-032-50831-3 (pbk)
ISBN: 978-1-003-39985-8 (ebk)

DOI: 10.4324/9781003399858

Typeset in Galliard
by Apex CoVantage, LLC

Contents

Acknowledgements

We would like to acknowledge all members, past and present of the National Medical Schools Widening Participation Forum (NMSWPF) who have influenced this work for over a decade and will continue to do so for many years to come.

Authors

Samuel Adcock, University of Leicester, United Kingdom.

Louise Alldridge, Peninsula Medical School, University of Plymouth, United Kingdom and Griffith University Medical School, Gold Coast Queensland, Australia.

Glen Barry, Griffith University, Gold Coast, Queensland, Australia.

Robert Cartwright-Speakman, University of Manchester, Manchester, United Kingdom.

John Chilton, Peninsula Medical School, University of Plymouth, United Kingdom.

Sally Curtis, Faculty of Medicine, University of Southampton, United Kingdom.

Paul Garrud, Chair, Medical Schools Council Selection Alliance; Hon. Associate Professor, School of Medicine, University of Nottingham, United Kingdom.

Umair Gondal, University of Manchester, Manchester, United Kingdom.

Monisha Gupta, Final year medical student, University of Nottingham, United Kingdom.

Mandy Hampshire, Director of Undergraduate Medicine Admissions, Faculty of Medicine and Health Sciences, University of Nottingham, United Kingdom.

Enam Haque, Division of Medical Education, School of Medical Sciences, Faculty of Biology, Manchester University, United Kingdom.

Nadin Hawwash, Division of Medical Education, School of Medical Sciences, Faculty of Biology, Manchester University, United Kingdom.

Jacqueline Higham, Lancashire Teaching Hospitals NHS Foundation Trust, United Kingdom.

Michael House, Education Officer, Plymouth City Council, United Kingdom.

Sophie Hoyle, Student Access, Success and Development Officer, University of Manchester, United Kingdom.

Maxine Hughes, Formerly, Griffith University Medical School, Gold Coast Queensland, Australia.

Alex Jackson (RIP).

Albert Jennings, University of Manchester Medical School, United Kingdom.

Karen Johnstone, Peninsula Medical School, University of Plymouth, United Kingdom.

Andy Kardasz, Hull York Medical School, United Kingdom (Retired).

Sarah Kasher, Medicine Calling Project Manager at University of Leicester.

Jacquie Kelly, Faculty of Medicine, University of Southampton, United Kingdom.

Chloe Langford, Faculty of Medicine, University of Southampton, United Kingdom.

Peter Leadbetter, School of Medicine, Edge Hill University, United Kingdom.

Teleah Lindenberg, Formerly, Griffith University Medical School, Gold Coast Queensland, Australia.

Jono Madeley, Education Adviser, Plymouth City Council, United Kingdom.

Julie Monk, Peninsula Medical School, University of Plymouth, United Kingdom.

Danielle Nimmons, Department of Primary Care and Population Health, University College London, United Kingdom.

Ceri Nursaw, Consultant, Nursaw Associates, United Kingdom.

Clare Owen, Assistant Director, Medical Schools Council, Woburn House, London, United Kingdom.

Clare Ray, College of Medical and Dental Sciences Lead for Outreach and Widening Participation, University of Birmingham, United Kingdom.

Eliot L. Rees, School of Medicine, Keele University, Research Department of Primary Care and Population Health, University College London, United Kingdom.

Emily Róisín Reid, Director of Student Experience, Employability and Progression. Associate Professor, Unit for Social Sciences and Systems in Health, Division of Health Sciences, Warwick Medical School, Warwick University, United Kingdom.

Ben Ryan, Friarage Hospital, South Tees Hospitals NHS Foundation Trust, Northallerton, United Kingdom.

Nana Sartania, School of Medicine, College of Medical, Veterinary and Life Sciences, University of Glasgow, United Kingdom.

Karl Sweeney, Education Adviser, Plymouth City Council (2008–2015), Plymouth, United Kingdom.

Anjali Vaidyanathan, University of Manchester Medical School, United Kingdom.

Charlie Williams, University of East Anglia, United Kingdom.

Rachel Winter, University of Leicester, United Kingdom.

Series editor foreword

Our intention with this book series is to explore fresh approaches, highlight points of difference, and examine situations in which academics have sought to innovate around problems and develop more effective solutions to teaching future healthcare workers.

More specifically, we have taken this fresh approach partly in reference to the many clinical professions experiencing crises in recruitment. Central government responses to this have involved increasing school places or placing great emphasis on increasing staff health and well-being during core and foundation training. *Contemporary Pedagogies of Medicine and Health* focuses on innovation and good practice in relation to curriculum design and teaching. Books in the series are segmented into two core types.

1 Pedagogies of individual subjects taught as part of a curriculum

   - For example, Pedagogies for Biomedical Science

2 Pedagogies of topics or themes within clinical curriculums

   - For example, Pedagogies of Widening Participation

In addition to texts on individual curriculum areas, the series will include books on themes that might emerge in several areas across a curriculum – for example, introducing social justice concerns, ethics, or gender-related issues in medicine. A common feature of both formats is the variety of voices in chapters that create balanced monographs, which do not shy away from presenting differing stakeholder opinions or subjects. The series creates a space for critique and voicing of multiple points of view, which we believe are fundamental to drive forward meaningful progress in curriculum development. To this end, we welcome works co-authored with patients and students.

The international relevance of the series is driven by the fact that many problems in medical and healthcare education are consistent across borders (global), increasing recruitment, retention of staff, sustainable delivery, technological advancement, preservation of well-being, etc. As a result, the series content is highly internationally relevant because it focuses on concerns that transcend national boundaries. Similarly, innovations and new approaches are required in all locations to continue to deliver high-quality education.

Consequently, the need to develop pedagogy within healthcare education to facilitate changes in teaching clinical subjects is a pressing current concern. The Lancet Commission, in their report on medical education, opined that medical school curricula were currently not fit to meet societal demands and were *'outdated and static'*. This series offers a space for clinical tutors and academics to showcase how medical schools (and so curricula) can be made fit for the 21st century through the dissemination of evidence-based pedagogies for instruction, for which there is clearly a demand in terms of societal pressure but also a regulatory requirement.

The series' scope is broad and encourages submissions from underserved clinical subjects in terms of research and scholarship on education and pedagogy. We envisage cross-cutting themes in healthcare education and medical subjects but look to offer opportunities for specialisms that receive less limelight to showcase innovations, projects in allied healthcare and other clinical professions are very welcome. Moreover, there is scope for books to focus on new teaching methodologies present across different areas of medicine and other clinical subjects combined.

We believe this series will interest anyone involved in the development of healthcare professions because of the salience (and need) of education, workforce, and regulatory developments as we all attempt to increase the quantity and quality of trainees entering a health service.

Many registered professions suffer from issues regarding representation and diversity in their workforce, given the systemic barriers that applicants from non-traditional backgrounds can face. Formal efforts to rectify this originate in the late 1990s, with many different programmes now in place. A plethora of approaches and pedagogical techniques for teaching medical and healthcare students on this pathway have been created – reflecting the varied backgrounds of WP students. This wide-ranging multi-author publication brings together a substantial selection of case studies, methodologies, and practical examples for delivering WP courses reflective of this cohort's needs.

Louise Alldridge has brought to life a book that combines submissions from national policy leaders, globally renowned academics, and an international contributorship. This publication reflects the life cycle of teaching, not just higher education. It includes interventions required for primary and secondary school children as a form of engagement with medical career opportunities.

Almost no other books exist with an explicit focus on medicine and healthcare. Louise and her co-authors have created a go-to resource for any medical school or health faculty who wants to develop or expand their inclusive approach to education. Furthermore, it offers valuable advice on outreach methodologies to foster more representative recruitment for aspiring medical students still in school.

Preface

Following the publication of the 'Selecting for Excellence Final Report' (2014) by the Medical Schools Council, the drive to widen participation in Medicine increased significantly. The National Medical Schools Widening Participation Forum (NMSWPF) was, at this time, attended by Widening Participation Leads and focused mainly on increasing access to medicine for under-represented groups. Over the last ten years, the forum has expanded to a much larger organisation with subgroups and affiliations covering all aspects of widening participation, from access to success and progression. The membership now encompasses Medical and Clinical Educators, undergraduate and postgraduate students, and doctors at all stages of their training and careers. Our work shares and promotes best practice for widening participation at UK medical schools and acts as a problem-solving forum for widening participation leads.

The committee of the National Medical Schools Widening Participation Forum (NMSWPF) was approached to develop a book on Widening Participation in Medicine. The collective experience of the members of this forum, who are all leading practitioners across the spectrum of widening participation work, has been harvested to present the first evidence-based practical guide to pedagogies currently applied to Widening Participation in a medical setting. The chapters include case studies, research, and evaluation, drawing on the experiences and insights of a wide range of current Widening Participation practitioners from over half of the medical schools in the United Kingdom. National Leads on the Medical Schools Council, Education Specialist, and International WP champions are also key contributors to this book.

This comprehensive review and practical guide is presented in a cohesive way, following the medical student life cycle from Primary School to Practice. We highlight the different strategies that have been employed by medical schools to encourage, enable access to, and integrate students from under-represented backgrounds into the medical profession. The book draws on data and experience from existing initiatives to diversify undergraduate medical cohorts and the medical profession through case studies and examples of best practice in terms of widening participation that can be utilised by other medical schools or educators wishing to run similar initiatives.

Chapter 1

Introduction

Defining, deconstructing, and demystifying widening participation in medical education – national forum contribution

Louise Alldridge, Clare Ray, Enam Haque, Charlie Williams, Emily Róisín Reid, Mandy Hampshire, and Nana Sartania

Defining and redefining WP in a medical education setting

Defining widening participation is complex. John Blake, the director for Fair Access and Participation at the Office for Students stated at a recent conference that he did not like the phrase Widening Participation but instead preferred 'equality of opportunity'. This shift perhaps shows the deepening of understanding of the systemic barriers some students face in their journey to higher education. The Medical Schools Council defined Widening Participation as 'increasing the number of people from groups that have historically had a lower participation rate in medicine' (Medical Schools Council, 2014). This requires significant knowledge and understanding of which groups are under-represented and the multiple social, cultural, financial, and structural factors that construct this under-representation. By the time of publication of this book, the definitions will, most likely, have shifted once more. Universities new Access and Participation Plans call for each institution to define the 'Risk Indicators' that may impact prospective or current student 'successes' throughout the student life cycle, including access into higher education, continuation throughout the course, completion of the course, attainment of degree classification, and progression into work. The factors driving these risks and the barriers created need to be identified to enable their removal at all stages of the student journey, including aspiration building, selection, teaching and learning strategies, and careers beyond medical school.

This process of universities, or medical schools, identifying underlying risks to equality of opportunity allows for complexity to be embraced in all initiatives but individualised according to the local context. Widening Participation was created as a concept to address patterns of under-representation in Higher Education. However, it has different connotations in different settings and, more poignantly, different populations to target and assist in very complex personal

DOI: 10.4324/9781003399858-1

and social settings. Coastal and rural regions, for instance, could face different challenges than urban areas. Similarly, students who are care experienced or estranged could face different challenges to those with family at home to support applicants, and those in receipt of free school meals face financial and related social challenges not seen by those in financial stability. The process of addressing underlying risks involves not only identifying who is under-represented in the context of a programme but also understanding the reasons behind this under-representation. These undoubtedly include wider causal factors such as social structures, beliefs of key stakeholders, inclusive education and admissions policies, and economic influences. It requires us to look deeply into not only societal structures and beliefs but also the motives and visions of the institutions we serve, not least the medical schools and the medical profession.

In the context of Medicine, aspects of widening participation are undoubtedly complex and multifactorial. They include examining our own bias and expectations of how a 'medical student' should look, sound, and act. What makes a good medical student/doctor? Should all doctors share the same skills and characteristics, for example, a GP and a pathologist? We need to analyse 'who', in particular, is under-represented in the medical profession and why. We should also be considering each stage of medical education and the broad scope of this profession, not labelling characteristics, skills, and identities that may be specific to a narrow field of practice. We then need to understand how these expectations play out, in positive and negative ways, for students from a variety of backgrounds in our complex selection processes. Some contexts may not be predictive of good students, and others may be 'classed' in their expectations. For example, while contextual admissions are commonplace, there is still an over-reliance on traditional A-levels achieved at very high grades. Many medical schools still require candidates to pass entrance exams that are stacked in favour of those who can afford coaching and the fees required to register and to sit the examination. Many students who are privately educated also get help at their schools. In addition, what biases are played out in the interviews? A study by one of the authors, conducted ten years ago, analysed Medical Selection interviews at a UK medical school, through observation of interactions between candidates and interviewers with respect to different forms of class, gender, and race. They noted that when the candidate identity was similar to that of the interviewers, a more relaxed and encouraging interview was observed. Conversely, differences in class and culture between candidate and interviewer manifested in tension and sometimes discomfort for the interviewees. When talking about work experience, some interviewers were derogatory to those who worked in supermarkets and other non-clinical environments (unpublished data). Times have moved on, and most medical schools have transformed their selection to fairer scripted questions and scoring.

It is important to acknowledge that access to Medical School is also restrained by lack of income, for example, to finance UCAT (which is helped by bursaries) and GAMSAT exam fees or to pay for private coaching. In addition, travel costs to open days and interviews (helped by online interviews) are present another barrier for low-income families. Access to information and more importantly encouragement from peers/teachers/families can also be elusive. Some of these barriers can be partially alleviated by well-planned in-reach and outreach activities. In addition, WP students who manage to secure a place at medical school may have many overt and covert barriers to success, including 'misrecognition of talent' (Burke and McManus, 2011).

Hence, much consideration should be placed on what 'really' makes a good medical student and doctor and whether our access events, selection methods, and pedagogy consider the nuances of this talent in all backgrounds. In addition, can we ensure that we are targeting those that are most under-represented?

Moving onto success in medical school, what barriers do students face when it comes to exams, placements, commuting, working, accessing information, making friends, and even having food on campus that they can eat? Have we truly created an inclusive learning environment for all to thrive in their educational journey? For example, finance becomes a greater issue as students move onto the reduced finances of the NHS bursary. At this stage, many need to take up paid employment which impacts on their study time, friendships, and well-being. They may also feel that they do not 'fit in' and develop imposter syndrome. Success for these students is not all about passing assessments and graduating as a doctor.

Demystifying and deconstructing

Widening participation, in its current format, was an unknown entity amongst medical staff and students until recently. The key area of work that focused on the medical school experience of WP was the Medical Schools Council (MSC) Selecting for Excellence Final Report in 2014. This report identified the barriers for pupils from WP backgrounds from entering medical school and emphasised the need for targeted outreach in 'cold spot' regions of the UK. It also recognised the need for medical school-led access programmes, as well as considering contextual offers for pupils from WP backgrounds.

The National Medical Schools Widening Participation Forum (NMSWPF) was formed as a regional group in December 2015, after the founder (Dr Enam Haque) delivered a talk on widening participation to admissions leads in North West England. Following the talk, Dr Enam Haque invited those interested in collaborating on WP work to join him at a planning meeting at the University of Manchester. The forum expanded its reach beyond the North West the very next year and incorporated the perspectives from Wales and Scotland. With the expertise and guidance of colleagues, the group developed a constitution and terms of reference. They agreed that the focus would be on outreach activities, student access and admissions, as well as research on widening access. The organisation rapidly expanded to having a UK-wide footprint. Central to the expansion was the high-quality secretariat support provided by Helen Franklin, WP Manager at the University of Manchester, who ensured the efficient running of the organisation, maintaining member details, and organising biannual meetings and meetings with external parties.

A key principle of the NMSWPF, which continues to this day, was to provide an open platform for discussion and collaboration, sharing of expertise, and creating learning opportunities. With this approach, the group attracted academic and administrative staff from UK medical schools, as well as organisations involved in admissions and outreach. However, NMSWPF members quickly realised that a key stakeholder was missing from the meetings, the students. To address this, they appointed the first ever student lead (Michael Teixeira) in 2018 and they formed a national student working group. This group was tasked with delivering a medical schools conference on widening participation, funded, and organised by the MSC. This was delivered in London in November 2018, providing the opportunity for 100 staff and students to share their work and to network and explore new opportunities. The students, with the support of staff, have since organised six national WP conferences, including a remotely delivered 'WAMS Week' during the height of the Covid-19 pandemic in 2020. This was a series of online talks and workshops spread over a week in November, ensuring that even a pandemic would not prevent NMSWPF members from networking and sharing best practice.

The early years of the NMSWPF were a time of innovation and growth and helped to cement the foundations. This enabled the organisation to rapidly expand and begin to see the wider perspective of WP. The Forum, recognising the multifactorial contributions to fair access, progression, and success, has now formed subgroups to tackle key barriers in each of these areas. These subgroups have brought about collaborative work amongst the members from sharing good practice to research publications, ranging from access to medical school and beyond. All the contributors to this book are affiliated to the NMSWPF and document experiences of multiple aspects of WP (from primary schools through to the practice of medicine), here and overseas, through research, case studies, insights, and practical information.

Until we achieve better representation, there remains an urgent need to deconstruct narratives around widening access and participation. NMSWPF is a powerful collective which can innovate and advocate for alternative approaches to seeing significant transformative change within our lifetimes. As a result of significant effort, Medical Schools already have taken a range of steps from introducing Foundation Programmes to providing bespoke support to potential applicants to act as a proxy for economic, social, and cultural capital that helps them compete with applicants who come from more privileged backgrounds. We have moved beyond seeking equality (often termed 'meritocracy'), through policy interventions that are equally applied, such as 'robust' and 'fair' admissions processes. We are now achieving 'equity', where strategies like contextual admissions and widening access programmes serve to

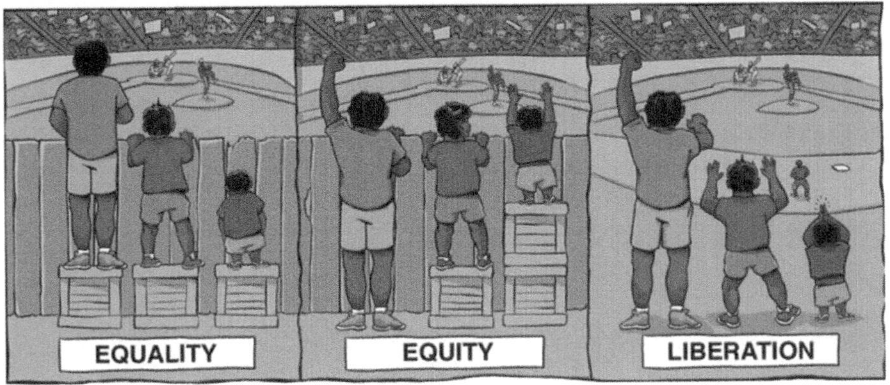

Figure 1.1 Equality, equity, and liberation

Image credit: Interaction Institute for Social Change | Artist: Angus Maguire interactioninstitute.org and madewithangus.com, respectively

level the playing field by acting as a proxy for the accumulation of parental/familial capital that these students might be missing. However, we must acknowledge that systemic barriers remain for candidates and institutions alike. Students continue to experience obstacles throughout their medical student careers and professional lifetimes, which have knock-on impacts on their career choices and destinations. As a collective, we need to take more radical interventions to meaningfully take down the barriers for these individuals (Figure 1.1). These are questions on which the forum will continue to reflect and act on in the future.

References

Burke, P. J., and McManus, J. (2011). Art for a few: Exclusion and misrecognitions in higher education admissions practices. *Discourses in Cultural Politics of Education*, 32(5), 699–712. doi: 10.1080/01596306.2011.620753
Medical Schools Council. (2014). *Selecting for Excellence Final Report*. www.medschools.ac.uk/media/1203/selecting-for-excellence-final-report.pdf

Chapter 2

The 'making connections' problem-based learning approach

Practicalities of supporting widening participation sixth formers

Andy Kardasz

Introduction and background

Hull York Medical School (HYMS) was founded in 2003 in response to the need to address the acute shortage of doctors, particularly GPs, within North Yorkshire, the Humber and North Lincolnshire, and Goole. Since its inception as a new medical school in the area, part of the HYMS philosophy is to run a variety of widening participation (WP) and fair access schemes across the region to help raise the aspirations of the students. Making Connections formed part of a portfolio of HYMS widening participation and fair access projects offered to schools and colleges. The idea for Making Connections was conceived out of the 'Gary project' set up in County Durham by Sarah Pearce. This project was aimed at raising the aspirations of some Year 10 pupils who were in danger of losing interest in science because of their predicted GCSE grades (Pearce and Gargett, 2005). The author in discussion with the then incumbent HYMS Widening Participation Officer (WPO) felt that with some modification of the Gary project, a Problem-Based Learning (PBL) approach using a number of so-called virtual patient scenarios based around topics studied at the post-16 level and followed by some appropriate hands-on physiology laboratory activities associated with the PBL scenarios could be offered to colleges and schools in the HYMS catchment area, particularly aimed at students who fulfilled the WP criteria.

Making Connections is a problem-based learning (PBL) approach to teaching post-16 biology to help students make a link between School science, Higher Education science, and science in the workplace. The PBL cases were chosen with A-level Biology and Advanced Health and Social Care curricula in mind. The term Making Connections aims to link topics covered in the PBL cases to the A-level Biology material covered at the six formers' institutions together as well as how to use with some relevant physiology activities undertaken at HYMS. Initially in 2005/6, Making Connections was set up as a project involving collaboration between HYMS, five sixth form colleges in Hull, Grimsby, Scunthorpe, Scarborough, York, and the local NHS facilities.

DOI: 10.4324/9781003399858-2

The teachers participated out of interest and commitment to a novel pedagogical approach. The teacher-facilitators at the various institutions received some training in PBL prior to the project's commencement. Students were given three different problem scenarios based around a so-called virtual patient. These scenarios presented a variety of topics linked to subject matter covered in their post-16 curricula. The topics included Asthma, Coronary heart disease, and Diabetes.

It was based on a five-week cycle of activities as shown in Table 1. In week 1, the students undertook a PBL session timetabled at their institutions as a double 1.5-hour lesson. The following week, week 2, the group shared the results of their research and discussed their learning with their facilitator. In week 3, the students undertook some web-based work and any further activity at the discretion of their facilitator. In week 4, the students visited HYMS and undertook some practical work associated with the appropriate PBL case that they had studied. In week 5, the students undertake a visit to their local hospital to visit an appropriate department associated with the topics they have studied in the relevant PBL case. In this case, it was the respiratory function laboratory, Scunthorpe Hospital, where the students undertook some respiratory function tests. However, due to staff shortages at the local hospital and difficulties in timetabling at the school/college, the visits to local NHS facilities were discontinued. In subsequent years, Making Connections was broadened out and offered to other colleges and schools in the HYMS region where students were particularly interested in studying medicine. The cycle of activities was shortened to a four-week period. The schools/colleges visited HYMS for either a morning or afternoon session and the activity included a PBL session followed by some practical work related to the PBL scenario. In the following discussion, the author will describe the practicalities of how using a

- **Week 1:**
- Presentation of case. The group formulates the learning outcomes and undertakes private study.
- **Week 2:**
- The group shares the results of their private study; the learning resources are identified and shared; tutor checks learning and may assess students.
- **Week 3:**
- The group undertakes a web-based research activity and any further work at the discretion of their facilitator.
- **Week 4:**
- Visit to HYMS to undertake a practical associated to the case.
- **Week 5:**
- Students visit different departments at their local hospital to gain an insight into those professions.

Figure 2.1 **The weekly cycle of activities**

PBL approach and appropriate hands-on physiology laboratory activities associated with the PBL scenarios, the readers can support WP students' learning.

Problem-Based Learning

Problem-Based Learning (PBL) was first developed in the late 1960s by Howard Barrows at McMaster University Medical School (Barrows and Tamblyn, 1976) and has subsequently been adopted by many medical schools throughout the world. PBL is a constructivist approach to learning, as well as being based on the principles of adult learning (Andragogy) (Kaufman, 2003). There is some confusion as to what is meant by the term PBL. One useful definition of PBL is that it is active learning stimulated by, and focused on a clinical, community, or scientific problem (Davis and Harden, 1999). In PBL, students are in a small group ideally containing no more than eight to ten students, together with a facilitator. The students are presented with triggers from a problem case (using a virtual patient) or a clinical scenario that is then used to define their own learning objectives (or outcomes) for that case. For those unfamiliar with PBL, here is a summary of the roles and responsibilities in a PBL group. The PBL facilitator guides the group learning by facilitating group discussion, helps the group to find appropriate depth and breadth of learning, oversees student interaction within the group, and attends to group dynamics for example. The facilitator should not provide easy answers to the group, collude with the group in bypassing the PBL process, persistently lead the discussion, and teach or give mini lectures. The role of the chair is to agree on the process for the group, introduce the cases for discussion, invite participation ensuring all group members are participating equally, stimulate discussion, and summarise and oversee timekeeping. The role of the scribe is to listen carefully to the discussion, note down all ideas and concepts, organise the notes clearly and creatively, check the accuracy of the notes taken, and contribute to the group discussion. The role of the student group member is to contribute as fully as possible; respect the roles of the scribe, chair, and facilitator and assist them in their roles; respect the contribution of other group members; and observe the shared group rules. The roles of the chair and scribe are rotated with each group so that every student in the group gets the opportunity to undertake these roles.

Once the group with the guidance of the facilitator have defined the learning outcomes for the case, they undertake independent, self-directed learning before they return as a group to share, discuss, and clarify their acquired knowledge (Wood, 2003). The idea of PBL is not to solve a problem but to use suitable problems to extend the students' knowledge and understanding. At HYMS, the guided discovery model of PBL is used, where the tutor has the learning outcomes and can with appropriate intervention guide the students towards the learning outcomes. At HYMS, the PBL sessions were modelled on the Maastricht 'seven jump' method (Wood, 2003). The stages are set out

> - Stage 1: read & comprehend problem, including clarification of terms.
> - Stage 2: state new problems & concepts to be studied.
> - Stage 3: brainstorm new problems & concepts.
> - Stage 4: arrive at provisional solutions.
> - Stage 5: set learning outcomes.
> - Stage 6: individuals & group engage in relevant study ensuring that all members cover complete set of learning outcomes.
> - Stage 7: group discuss and refine learning.

Figure 2.2 The PBL process used at HYMS adapted from the Maastricht 'seven jump method'

in Table 2. The problem is read out and the aim is to identify a problem or problems and clarify any terms, define the key concepts identified, brainstorm ideas and reach some interim solutions, discuss key learning outcomes, research these and share this information with each other at subsequent sessions. The students research all the learning outcomes, rather than splitting them up amongst the group and each student investigating just one outcome. As mentioned above, the tutor is present to guide the students so that they stay on track with the learning outcomes.

For a further explanation of the PBL process and how to undertake it, the reader is directed to articles by Davis and Harden (1999) and Wood (2003).

Student allocation

The HYMS Widening Participation Officer (WPO) contacted schools and colleges in the HYMS region particularly those institutions where many of the students fulfilled some or most of the indicators of a non-traditional Higher Education (HE) background, such as attendance at a low-performing school (both in attainment and progression to HE), in receipt of Educational Maintenance Allowance, having no parental experience of HE.

Each college or school selected eight to ten students studying at post-16 level by open application to make up a PBL group. As previously mentioned, ideally a PBL group should not contain more than eight to ten students, but in practice groups still work efficiently with 12 students. Students were studying A-levels in science subjects, Advanced Health and Social Care, or a combination of the two. The tutors (or Facilitators) were usually Biology teachers who were chosen by the colleges and schools based on their interest in teaching and a willingness to participate in the project.

The PBL session

In the initial years of Making Connections, the sessions were run as follows: Each PBL group consisted of eight to ten students and a tutor (or facilitator).

A session typically lasts 1.5 hours (or a double lesson) and was timetabled as part of their enhancement studies. The group elects a chair and a scribe for each session to record the discussion. These roles are rotated at each session so that members of the group can undertake these roles. Students were given some induction into undertaking a PBL session. The induction consisted of an explanation of the roles of the chair, scribe, members of the group, and the facilitator. In addition, an explanation of the steps involved in a PBL session to generate the learning outcomes for each case was given to the students. Initially in this project, the author visited the institutions and ran an extended PBL session with a scenario explaining the PBL session so that both students and facilitators understood the process. To aid in learning how to do PBL, the author produced a handout that explained the various roles in a PBL group, as well as the PBL process.

Setting up

In later years, the programme was changed such that schools and colleges were invited to visit HYMS in week 4. The process was modified and the HYMS WPO recruited current medical students to undertake the PBL process, as well as assist in the practical work. Years 1 and 2 students, and when available students from Years 3 and 4 (acting as student ambassadors (SAs)) were given the roles of facilitators and scribes. However, it would be better not to use Year 1 students in their initial term at medical school as they will yet not be so familiar with the PBL process. By term 2, these Year 1 students will be more conversant with the PBL process. Prior to the school/college visiting, usually a couple of hours before the visit, a brief meeting is held with the SAs, and all the activities explained. Generally, there were often up to 40 visiting students, and so we tended to recruit eight medical students as SAs. In the author's experience, some visiting students in the PBL groups will feel self-conscious and be quiet during the session. When undertaking the briefing to the SAs before the visit, do remind them to try and engage any quiet students during the session. As your WPO should know how many students will be visiting on the day, you can allocate pairs of SAs to a group of students and a room that will be used. Assign one SA to be the facilitator and the other to be the scribe.

Each group of visiting students together with their student ambassadors were allocated to PBL rooms; it is important to make sure that you have enough rooms available in your institution to accommodate small groups of up to 14 persons. The rooms should have a large enough table and chairs for the groups to sit around, preferably in view of the whiteboard or screen. In addition, the rooms should have whiteboards available to allow the scribe to record relevant points from the group's discussion, as well as to list the learning outcomes that they have proposed. Do ensure that the rooms have sufficient marker pens for the groups to use. It is useful to also have a copy of a medical dictionary to hand. Moreover, you should have sufficient copies of the scenario to give to the visiting students, as well as the SAs; do make sure that the SAs' copies include the learning outcomes. However, if you have rooms equipped with a large screen coupled to a computer, then you can project the scenario on screen. If you have the time and resources available, such as a video camera and a simulated patient (SP), you could show a video of a consultation with the SP. Once the visiting schools/colleges have arrived and been welcomed, they were given an introduction to the day's events, before being divided up into groups and sent off to the PBL rooms with their allocated SAs.

Generally, the groups would be allocated around 40–45 minutes to undertake a scenario based on a virtual patient. Timekeeping is important, so someone must oversee the overall running of the outreach sessions; usually visiting schools and colleges are at the medical school for a limited period. Once the groups have completed the PBL, you can then get the groups to undertake a variety of practical activities. In the case of HYMS, the writer had planned for the students to carry out some practical physiology work related to the PBL scenario. The type of activities the students undertake depends upon what equipment is available at your institution. At HYMS, we were able to offer students the opportunity to undertake physiological work using the ADInstruments PowerLab data acquisition system. Using this equipment, we can get students to undertake such things as ECGs, static and dynamic lung function, breathing rates, as well as nerve conduction velocity depending upon the scenario planned for use. See below for more details of the practical work.

The scenarios

When writing a scenario, it is important to bear in mind what facilities and equipment you have at your institution. I would recommend if possible, liaising with the heads of biology at local schools/colleges that you intend to target to discuss what would be useful to include as topics for scenarios so that you can write learning outcomes that encompass the aims and objectives of the post-16 curricula that students have covered at their institution. If this is not possible, and if you know what examining board(s) the schools/colleges are using, such as AQA or OCR, for example, these can be accessed online. The author had access to a range of biology titles that comprised part of the Cambridge Modular Sciences series for A- and AS-level Biology that was used to choose some topics that matched equipment that HYMS had readily available. Using clinically based scenarios is definitely a good way to stimulate the students. Additionally, the learning outcomes can be used to enable the students to revise some subject topics they have covered as part of their post-16 study at their institutions, as well as introduce a few concepts that can stretch them intellectually and give them an awareness of some of the study matter as part of the undergraduate medicine curriculum. I would aim to have no more than five or six learning outcomes for a case. Contingent on what you wish the students to experience in a PBL session, the outcomes should be written utilising the three domains (Cognitive, Affective, and Psychomotor) of Bloom's Taxonomy appropriate to the topic that the scenario comprises (Bloomstaxonomy.net). The learning outcomes may just encompass the bio-medical, psychosocial, or evidence-based ones, or it can be a combination of all three. This will depend upon factors such as what equipment, facilities, and at what point in their programme of study your SAs have reached, as well as what insight of studying medicine you wish the visiting students to experience.

In Table 3, this is an example of a scenario called Elizabeth Little, together with some of the associated learning outcomes. As you can see, there are signs and symptoms of Asthma, as well as the results of some respiratory tests. The problem scenario contains cues (or triggers) in the scenario to guide the

---

Name: Elizabeth Little
Age: 16 years
Gender: Female
Height: 1.60m
Occupation: Student in year 11 at a local comprehensive school.
Social situation: Lives with parents and 18-year-old brother.
Elizabeth comes to see you complaining of wheezing, cough, and a tight chest. On questioning her, she tells you that these symptoms appeared to have begun a few weeks ago and get worse at night and in the early morning. Her wheezy breathing can clearly be heard. She is concerned that the symptoms are interfering with her enjoyment of playing sport.
You arrange for her to have some lung function tests. Her Peak Expiratory Flow Rate (PEFR) was measured by a mini-Wright Peak flow meter, which showed a low value in comparison to the norm expected for her age and height (399L/min ± 85 L/min). Spirometry was performed and demonstrated that her FEV1 is some 30% reduced compared to the norm for her age (3.12L).

You discuss the results with her and explain the treatment and management of her condition.

The learning outcomes identified for Elizabeth Little.

Problem: Asthma

The learning outcomes for this session from this patient are

- The structure of the respiratory tract
- Lung volumes and capacities
- The causes of asthma
- Simple lung function tests; PEFR and Spirometry and relationship to asthma.

Figure 2.3 An example of a PBL scenario and some of the learning outcomes

students to stimulate discussion. Some of the group may recognise some of the signs and symptoms as Asthma, either they suffer from it themselves, or a sibling or school friend does, and they may well tell the group. In the author's experience, this will activate their prior knowledge and you will no doubt get a range of responses from the students. Here, the SA acting as facilitator can pose a question or two to the group to generate some responses and encourage the students to make some suggestions. Regarding the respiratory tests, again, some of the group may know a little about this from their own experience and thus will be able to inform the group, or if not, then the SA facilitator can direct them with appropriate hints. The SAs will be well adept at the PBL process, encourage the group by posing questions to the group, and generate some discussion of their thoughts. At the end of this session, if the groups have generated some learning outcomes, that is fine, but if they haven't, that is also okay as they will have experienced a taster of what it is like to participate in a PBL session. Overall, over the years that the author has been involved in such sessions, the students have engaged in the PBL process. However, you will probably find the odd student or two in a group that will remain quiet in the session or contribute very little to the discussion. Sometimes some students are initially shy to say something, but generally as the session progresses, they feel more confident to participate in the discussion. Feedback from both staff and students has been very positive. The scenarios have worked very well, and the students have engaged enthusiastically with the material and related activities.

Practical example

The practical session planned that was associated with the scenario Elizabeth Little was based on the students undertaking a shortened version of a HYMS Year 1 respiratory physiology practical. All the groups convened in the physiology teaching lab, where the author gave a brief introduction to the practical with the aims and outcomes of the session, as well as a short overview of the rationale of respiratory function tests and measurement of lung volumes and capacities. The students in groups of three or four with two SAs to help were allocated to a PowerLab station. Each station was comprised of a desktop computer (with a keyboard and monitor) coupled to an ADInstruments PowerLab connected to a flow head. In addition, at each station, there were several Mini-Wright peak flow meters together with the peak expiratory flow charts showing the normal values.

In each group of visiting students, usually in groups of three or four, one of them agreed to be the subject and sign a consent form to undertake the practical and the signed consent form was then kept by the visiting school/college teacher. All the students in each group were given a copy of the practical protocol. Once the spirometer had been calibrated for each subject in each group, the students aided by the SAs first measured lung volumes, such as tidal volume, and inspiratory and expiratory reserve volumes, before calculating various lung capacities. The PowerLab software allows users to measure and calculate volume, etc. from the displays on the monitor. Once these initial activities had been undertaken, the groups then progressed onto undertaking some pulmonary function tests. The subjects inhaled maximally and then exhaled as forcefully and fully as possible (that is, inhale as much as possible and then exhale until no more air can be expired). The spirometer data window displayed both peak inspiratory and peak expiratory flow, and from the data window they could calculate their forced vital capacity (FVC) and forced expiratory volume in one second (FEV1) and then calculate their FEV1/FVC ratios. In addition, the students were then shown by the SAs how to correctly use the Mini-Wright peak flow meters and recorded their peak flow and compared their readings with the peak expiratory flow charts showing the normal values. At the end of the session, generally in the last 10–15 minutes, the students were brought together for a round-up of the session. It is useful to have a short question-and-answer session. You can ask the whole of the group, or one can get the students into groups of three or four depending on the numbers and then pose a question and give them a minute or so to discuss the answer and then go around each group. To end the session, a brief summary of what they have undertaken is given. The students can take away the practical session protocol.

Alternatives

If your institution doesn't have any PowerLabs or similar equipment, you can still undertake some sort of practical session with them depending on the scenario and the outcomes, you have set. With the above respiratory scenario, if you have any handheld spirometers, you could undertake the dynamic spirometry with them. Or just use the Mini-Wright peak flow meters. If not, then you could undertake a brief introduction to a respiratory examination, or just allow to listen for the various breath sounds, for example, with stethoscopes.

Discussion

In these sessions, students are interacting with medical students and are getting a small taste of what it is like to be a medical student. Talking to the SAs, they can gain some valuable insight into studying medicine and certainly the feedback from such sessions has been positive. One of the most important things to take into consideration is that these visiting students are getting an opportunity to experience one aspect of studying medicine. In these sessions, the medical students acting as SAs can provide an insight into life as a medical student, and act as a role model, as well as engaging students who, prior to the visit, may not have considered studying medicine. Anecdotally, the sixth formers found their participation useful in giving them insight into areas of

Biology, it allowed them to hone their research skills, and it gave them an introduction to teaching and learning methods in higher education and relating the theory and application of science. In addition, they felt that their participation strengthened and refined their decision to apply for medical school.

Using medical students to facilitate WP programmes as SAs confer many benefits to the students themselves. Ylonen (2010, 2012) identified the experience of being a mentor as financially rewarding, as well as developing their CV, improving their self-confidence, communication skills, and their teaching ability and their altruism. Similarly, in a recent 'quick glance' study, Haque et al. (2021) reported that medical student ambassadors improved their own learning, with increased knowledge in different subject areas, as well as improved their teaching and self-confidence. Individual students commented that their confidence had increased, and that they were more focused on their learning and were pleased to find that they were able to meet the intellectual demands of the WP sessions. Utilising a PBL approach in which appropriate scenarios and outcomes aligned to the post-16 curriculum with associated practical work can allow the WP students the opportunity to temporarily become medical students for a short period and gain an awareness of some of the learning and teaching methods employed in studying medicine.

References

Barrows, H. S., and Tamblyn, R. M. (1976). An evaluation of problem-based learning in small groups utilising a simulated patient. *Journal of Medical Education*, 51, 51–54.

Bloom's Taxonomy [Online]. www.bloomstaxonomy.net (accessed 24 August 2023)

Davis, M. H., and Harden, R. M. (1999). AMEE medical education guide N0.15: Problem-based learning: A practical guide. *Medical Teacher*, 21(2), 130–140.

Haque, E., Kardasz, A., and Alldridge, L. (2021). What impact does teaching in outreach activities have on medical students' own learning and teaching skills? A pilot study. *Widening Participation and Lifelong Learning*, 23(2), 152–163.

Kaufman, D. M. (2003). ABC of learning and teaching in medicine: Applying educational theory in practice. *British Medical Journal*, 326, 213–216.

Pearce, S. J., and Gargett, A. (2005). You be the doctor-solve Gary's problem: Using problem-based learning at school to raise aspirations for medicine and other science-based NHS careers. *Clinical Teacher*, 2(1), 49–51.

Wood, D. F. (2003). ABC of learning and teaching in medicine: Problem based learning. *British Medical Journal*, 326, 328–330.

Ylonen, A. (2010). The role of student ambassadors in higher education: An uneasy association between autonomy and accountability. *Journal of Further and Higher Education*, 34(1), 97–104.

Ylonen, A. (2012). Student ambassador experience in higher education: Skills and competences for the future? *British Educational Research Journal*, 38(5), 801–811.

Chapter 3

Embedding widening participation in the medical curriculum

Louise Alldridge, Julie Monk, John Chilton, Michael House, Jono Madeley, Karl Sweeney, and Karen Johnstone

Introduction and background

'Doctors as Educators' is a longitudinal Special Study Unit (SSU) undertaken by all undergraduate medical students at Peninsula Medical School as an integral part of their curriculum. SSUs are components of Student Selected Components introduced by the GMC. Over the course of an academic year, students work in groups, supported by an expert facilitator, to create a resource communicating information about a healthcare issue to a specified demographic. Students develop core professional skills, including teamwork, communication, reflection to prepare them for a lifelong role informing and listening to the public, and training and mentoring future healthcare colleagues.

The Medical School, in partnership with Plymouth City Council's Department of Education, Participation and Skills (EPS), piloted a project within this SSU. The projects aimed to highlight and address key aspects of Widening Participation (WP) and the health consequences of poverty and inequality. The challenges here were to adapt the SSU to incorporate WP (through building aspirations), promote health and well-being to schoolchildren, and trigger a change in attitudes of staff and current students regarding WP.

The medical students were tasked to produce and deliver a variety of inspirational and aspirational outreach activities in primary and secondary schools. These were designed to be sustainable learning and teaching resources for the schools and for our WP outreach at Peninsula Medical School. The resources produced aimed to convey messages of well-being and healthy lifestyle promotion alongside developing a positive mindset to achieve at school and a 'for me' attitude towards a career in medicine. The activities were – and many still are – delivered in schools by our Widening Access to Medicine Society (WAMS) in primary and secondary schools with a high proportion of pupils from an educationally and socially disadvantaged background.

The Widening Participation element continues to be a key component of the Doctors as Educators SSU. Furthermore, this project is used as a stepping stone to develop the skills and behaviours necessary for the SSU in the

DOI: 10.4324/9781003399858-3

following year which centres on creative approaches to advocacy for well-being and has students working directly alongside local community groups. We include examples of resources used by our own student outreach team and in the primary and secondary schools (Table 3.1) and discuss the challenges, development, benefits, and impact of embedding WP in the curriculum through incorporation in the SSU.

Sharing a vision: meeting a requirement

Prior to the conception of the project, the Conservative government had overhauled the existing National Curriculum, minimising the extent to which it was centrally prescribed and theoretically allowing schools freedom to develop their own curricula. Overall, the philosophy was to redesign the education system to maximise the long-term benefit to the UK economy of more technically and scientifically qualified future workers and administrators (Granoulhac, 2018). The policy included a 'forensic focus' (a term commonly used by Ofsted) on literacy, numeracy, and the sciences, the redefinition of the curriculum as a body of knowledge to be passed on to younger generations (Stone, 2017), and the encouragement, via substantial financial incentives, of schools to opt out of Local Authority control and become Academies or Free Schools. As a consequence, the school curriculum became decentralised and newly created schools were free to teach any curriculum they wished, beyond the 'basics' of English, Maths, Science, and PE. This resulted in pressure to reduce and even remove 'non-traditional' subjects like Personal Social Health and Economic Education (PSHEE) and Citizenship from already busy school timetables so schools could devote more time to improve English, Maths, and Science grades. None of these reforms were applied then (nor now) to the private sector of education, from where a disproportionate number of medical students and the political class in the UK are derived (Sutton Trust, 2019).

Alongside these reforms, from 2011 onwards, it was decided to discontinue a highly successful and very popular National Healthy Schools Award programme. This scheme was a well-funded, high-quality, and effective means of promoting health education across all schools. This programme centred on developing pupils' understanding of how to keep physically healthy, eat healthily, and maintain an active lifestyle. In addition, extracurricular activities aided the development of pupils' age-appropriate understanding of healthy relationships (Ofsted, 2022). These wide-ranging cutbacks to publicly funded bodies and programmes were part of 'austerity' measures and a clear indication that Health Education/Healthy Lifestyles was no longer regarded as a high-priority subject or a statutory part of the National Curriculum. Schools therefore needed to find alternative ways to ensure local children were equipped with the knowledge of how to stay healthy and form healthy relationships. The loss of such a vital element of education had far-reaching consequences for the health and well-being of children and disproportionately for children from lower socio-economic areas (Milburn, 2012). Furthermore, these 'cuts' had the potential to increase the burden on the NHS. It was clear that this education needed to be maintained for the benefit of the school children and our future healthcare providers.

In 2013, the Department for Education (DfE) introduced non-statutory guidance for Personal, Social, Health and Economic Education (PSHEE) which has been periodically reviewed and updated (UK Government, 2013). The emergence of PSHEE into the curriculum had the potential for schools to develop and implement an evidence-based, needs-led approach to health and well-being education that reflected actual developmental needs of children and young people. However, many schools and their teachers were and continue to be overburdened, and a non-statutory addition to the curriculum was understandably overlooked, particularly in schools with larger numbers of children in poverty, majority of whom were potentially most in need of the sessions. Despite being non-statutory, schools were still held accountable via regular Office for Standards in Education (Ofsted) inspections which included an Outcome regarding 'the extent to which pupils adopt healthy lifestyles' to be taken into consideration. Thus, the development of PSHEE policy and curriculum in this setting paved the way for much-needed collaboration between education, health, and community-based sectors. It was with this backdrop that a long-term partnership between Plymouth City Council's Citizenship, Health and Wellbeing Team, and Peninsula Medical School was founded. Through this partnership, Peninsula Medical School gained insight and access to schools with a high proportion of pupils from Widening Participation backgrounds. The ensuing outreach events gave schools access to personal, social, and health education alongside aspiration-building sessions delivered by medical students who embodied Widening Participation and the reality of what can be attained for pupils from similar backgrounds as themselves.

It is also worth noting that at the time of writing this remains the case to an extent – although Relationships and Sex Education is now a statutory requirement across all state schools. Also, health education in general is now given slightly more prominence forming as it does, a part of the 'Personal Development' judgement within the current Inspection Framework.

Partnership development: 2013

The key objectives of Peninsula Medical School, Plymouth City Council, and local schools and pupils in Plymouth were inextricably linked and forming a partnership was clearly mutually beneficial. Whilst Plymouth City Council's Citizenship, Health and Wellbeing Team's key objective was the promotion of high-quality health education in all primary and secondary schools in the city, there was a national push to widen participation in elite programmes such as medicine from the Government's Social Mobility and Child Poverty Report (Milburn, 2012) and the Selecting for Excellence Report (Medical Schools

Council, 2014). Implementation of extensive and sustained outreach to raise awareness of the possibilities of a career in medicine as a real proposition was and still is required, but with few resources and time.

Peninsula Medical School had recently developed a new Primary School to Practice Widening Participation Strategy called Peninsula Pathways to Healthcare Professions (PPHP) which incorporates a longitudinal sustained strategy to build aspirations and instil a 'can do' and 'for me' attitude in pupils from an early age. The PPHP aimed to help children from under-represented backgrounds to view a medical career as a reality from the age of 5 and sustain and develop support through to UCAS application, UCAT examination, and medical selection interviews. The Widening Access to Medical School (WAMS) programme (medical students who deliver outreach events) was, and remains, an important aspect of this strategy. Discussions between the Head of Plymouth City Council Education Directorate and the Medical School WP Lead were followed by meetings with the Education Leads for PSHEE. It was evident that a mutually beneficial project could be initiated in schools in the most deprived areas of Plymouth to combine building aspirations and life chances alongside conveying important messages of health and well-being.

Many head teachers in Plymouth understood the importance of health education at the time, despite its diminution, as their schools were (and still are in most cases) in areas of high unemployment, high crime, intergenerational benefits dependency, and negative health outcomes (Plymouth City Council, 2012). These schools were particularly keen to engage with the support offered by the Council to implement non-statutory Personal Social Health and Economic (PSHE) Education. This included topics such as drugs education, relationships (including online) and sex education, the importance of physical activity and diet for a healthy lifestyle, mental and emotional health and well-being, and risk management. Peninsula Medical School, keen to increase interest in and access to Medicine as a career for those from under-represented demographics, joined ranks and sessions were developed and delivered by medical students to pupils from a Widening Participation background through the Doctor as Educator Student Selected Component (SSC) across Plymouth.

Introducing widening participation in the medical and local primary and secondary school curriculum

As a professional degree programme, education of all medical students in the UK is aligned to the General Medical Council's (GMC) Outcomes for Graduates (GMC, 2020). The outcomes set the standards for medical education and training as well as defining the knowledge, skills, and attributes required by newly qualified doctors and as such form the basis for curricula, assessment, and regulation.

The GMC first introduced the Student Selected Component (SSC) into the medical curricula to enable students to engage and complete projects that were additional to the core curriculum. These projects aimed to help students demonstrate specific learning objectives and skills through independent and collaborative educational activities and research. Doctors as Educators spans the academic year, which enables them to develop the skills, attitudes, and practices of a competent teacher. Outcomes for Graduates recognises that doctors have a responsibility to educate and mentor other doctors and members of the multidisciplinary team, as well as patients, care workers, and relatives. Doctors as Educators aims to provide students with an understanding of medical education while developing skills and confidence to facilitate learning by creating a teaching and learning resource. When the module was first introduced, students were encouraged to choose to educate diverse target audiences including patients, the public, medical students, and schools.

This particular Doctors as Educators project was introduced at a Teachers Education Conference organised by Plymouth City Council by the WP Lead at the medical school. The project received a lot of interest and was subsequently discussed with the SSU leads at the medical school. Both parties recognised that the SSU presented an ideal opportunity to deliver the dual goals of Plymouth City Council and Peninsula Medical School in target schools and the benefits of combining PSHEE education and aspiration building. Medical students were supported to develop and deliver meaningful age-appropriate educational resources and activities to promote health and well-being in schools in areas of poverty, inequality, and poorer health and well-being. In addition, the medical students conveyed messages of aspiration to achieve at school and the realistic prospect of a career in medicine. It was also anticipated that WP activities could trigger a change in attitudes towards WP not only amongst school students but also amongst teachers. In order to achieve 'buy-in' from the medical students, the authors ran workshops within the SSU to promote the importance of WP and health and well-being in schools with high proportion of underprivileged pupils. Students who elected to do the school-based projects attended sessions run by our partner PSHEE educators to enable them to deliver meaningful age-appropriate educational and inspirational outreach activities. Projects for older pupils included help to gain access to 'privileged' information and advice regarding navigation of the complex selection and admissions processes for medical school. Such information and practical resources are available in private schools and at cost through private organisations whose fees are out of reach for many pupils from under-represented backgrounds.

Every year the students produced a comprehensive collection of widening participation resources, underpinned by scholarship and 'trialed' on primary and secondary students and their teachers. Many of these resources are still being used ten years later as tools to promote healthy living, build aspirations, and instil the reality of a career in Medicine (see Table 3.1 for examples).

Table 3.1 Selected examples of the types of activities and resources designed by students, many of which are still used in our widening access programme

	Target group	*Resource*	*Sustainability*
Teddy bear hospital	Primary	Bring your soft toy to the doctor and get a 'pawscription' followed by educational and aspirational activities	Running for over ten years as a WAMS resource and continues to be a mainstay of primary outreach work
Basic life support, Dr ABC, choking, epilepsy	Primary and secondary	Many students developed emergency first-aid scenarios and resources used in schools and more widely	Basic life support and emergency first aid were also a core focus of junior skills for life event organised by Plymouth City Council for Year 6 students
Health and well-being	Primary and secondary	Many students have developed resources aimed at promoting health and well-being (including hand hygiene, Bharata dancing, self-care and resilience, mindfulness, healthy eating, physical activity)	A number of these are still used as WAMS resources
Applying to medical school calendar	Secondary	An 18-month calendar with key events in the application process and links to resources and aspirational advice	Published for a number of years and circulated through WAMS and Peninsula Pathways
Preparation for MMIs and UCAT	Secondary	Videos	Used by WAMS and Peninsula Pathways and on social media

Challenges

Loss of health education in primary and secondary schools

The project was initiated due to the loss of statutory 'Health Education/ Healthy Lifestyles' education in schools. This loss presented a major challenge

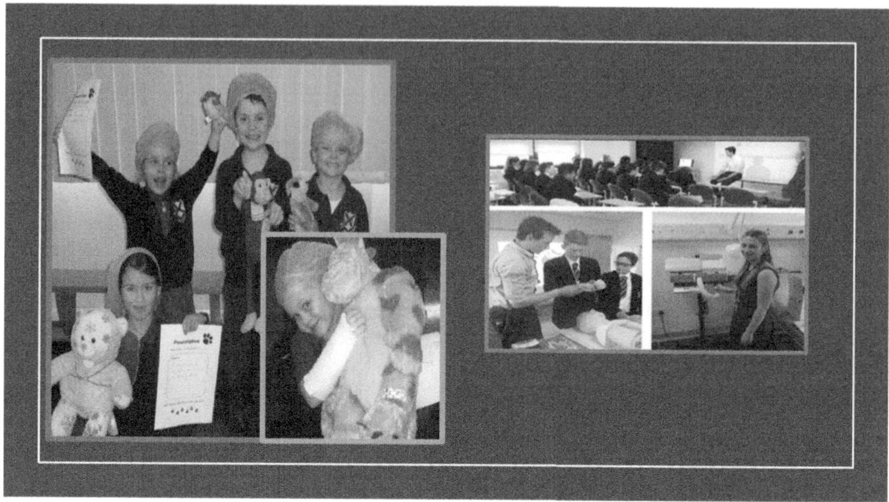

Figure 3.1 Illustration of in-reach and outreach activities 'in action' that were designed and delivered by students and remain part of our Widening Participation Outreach today, ten years later

for teachers who were invested in and supported pupil health and well-being. With little room in the curriculum and already overstretched teaching staff, it was a concern that something as vital as health education was not going to be delivered. The far-reaching challenges of this included declining health and well-being as well as 'unhealthy' behaviour in children of a vulnerable age and disposition. Knock on affects for education and already overburdened health-care services could also be seen as future challenges.

Changes in school staff and demographics

Local primary and secondary schools are monitored with regard to pupil social demography including free school meals (FSM) eligibility, English as an additional language, ethnicity as well as school characteristics such as class sizes. Staff turnover in schools can also be a challenge. The positioning of our partners as education specialists for PCC facilitated contacts with current staff and information regarding the demography of the pupils, to ensure we were targeting schools with higher proportion of pupils on free school meals.

Access to schools

One of the key challenges for achieving Widening Participation is identifying and gaining access to schools with a high proportion of pupils from lower socio-economic backgrounds. In addition, these schools were dealing with competing needs of their pupils and finding the time to host medical students was particularly difficult. These challenges were instantly overcome through our connections with PCC who identified the schools that were most in need and with highest proportion of children from Widening Participation Backgrounds. Initial meetings were held between Peninsula School of Medicine WP Lead and the Head Teachers, and the schools subsequently welcomed the projects and the chance to have medical students lead sessions.

Appropriate content and level for different age groups

Designing and delivering content at an appropriate level and depth for pupils of different ages and particularly with sensitive content was a major challenge for both the students and the academics, who are trained in post-18 medical education. These specific challenges were negated by expert sessions delivered by PSHEE Leads. Over the subsequent years, the PSHEE Leads ensured all educational resources developed by students were relevant, contemporary, and age-appropriate. Interestingly, statutory relationships and sex education has recently been discussed in the media due to opposition from groups to its inclusion in schools (BBC report, 2023).

Once students had selected to focus their SSU project on WP and Health and Wellbeing, members of the PCC PSHE advisory team facilitated interactive workshops covering educational theory, lesson plan design and delivery, engaging students in the classroom, and checking understanding. The PCC education leads were also available to check lesson plans and learning outcomes, and answer any questions to consolidate understanding of the needs of the 'audience'. This session and further input over the module enabled the medical students to produce excellent, contemporary, and sustainable resources.

Engaging school-aged children

A further challenge was to ensure that our medical students were well equipped to engage a class of primary or secondary school pupils and covey the key messages. In the first session of the module, the education leads for WP, the 'Doctors as Educators' module, and Plymouth City Council's Citizenship, Health and Wellbeing Team delivered a plenary to the entire year group. This session outlined the value and necessity of WP in the diversification of the medical profession and aimed to develop student understanding of the health and well-being needs of children in the participating schools. Examples of previous successful creative and innovative projects were also included to inspire the medical students to opt for a WP/health and well-being based project.

Developing an understanding of effective pedagogical methods for teaching and learning about health education was a challenge for some medical students. The observation from council officers responsible for providing teacher training was that students who had experienced a more traditional, didactic approach to learning were less comfortable with pluralistic, pupil-centred lesson planning and delivery methods.

Who elected to do a WP project and cultural opposition?

We welcomed and encouraged a broad demographic of medical students to take up these WP projects. The school-based WP projects, however, were almost entirely selected by medical students from a WP background and/or current members of WAMS. Although this is advantageous regarding role modelling for the school students and sustainability within the WAMS network, an impactful educational, social, and cultural experience for those from more privileged backgrounds, who may be less familiar with the social and health issues in the schools, was missed. Engaging medical students from more privileged backgrounds remains a challenge and students from WP backgrounds still dominate in the uptake of these projects.

There was also overt opposition from some of the students from more privileged backgrounds who had dissimilar cultural, social, and political backgrounds to the widening participation students and subsequently held different beliefs and values. Some of these students were sadly not only disinterested, dismissive, and even discourteous about the projects but also voiced unwanted comments during the introductory session of the SSU. Fortunately, there were a core of students from WP backgrounds who were aware of the barriers to accessing medicine and also the social and economic determinants of health and well-being, who opted for the WP projects, conversely those students from a traditional background missed a key, and much needed, social educational opportunity.

In more recent years, the introduction of a Foundation to Medicine Programme, as an alternative entry to medicine at this Medical School and introduction of a team-based project within the SSU have continued to have a positive impact on this issue. Students are no longer formally educated about WP through the SSU, but WP remains a key target for projects. Informal education on the challenges faced by WP students takes place through small group sessions, driven by students from WP backgrounds, particularly those coming through the Foundation Programme. This results in students, from more privileged backgrounds, inevitably being involved in WP projects championed by students from WP backgrounds, increasing the understanding of challenges faced by young people from a WP background.

Autonomy of WAMS

WAMS is an independent society and the committee has the final say on what resources/activities they deliver. As medical students, they have limited time and often do not have the time to train students to deliver new resources. Consequently, despite the creativity and potential of many student SSU projects, only a select few have been sustained as WAMS resources.

Duality of the sessions: combining WP and health and well-being messages

Additional challenges included combining aspirational messages along with those of health and well-being. This was achieved in most cases, even if subliminally through delivery by medical students from similar background and in some cases by former pupils at the schools they delivered too. However, the dual message did not always come across, and consequently some sessions were designed solely as Widening Access resources, particularly those for older school pupils.

Sustainability

Following the success of the pilot study, the widening participation continues to be a fixture in the Doctors as Educators module to this day. Sustainability of the resources produced has been a challenge as medical students move on to the next stage of a very intense programme. Many projects remained 'one-offs', although as mentioned earlier, remarkably some of the resources are still being used today, ten years later, as outreach tools through our Peninsula Pathways to Medicine and WAMS (Widening Access to Medical School) and are included in Box 1 and illustrated in Box 2. One of the biggest influences on sustainability of the resource was the 'drive' of the student creator. Medical students are time poor; the curriculum is demanding with competing modules and continuous assessment. For most students, once the SSU was complete, they understandably move on to and become immersed in the next module and concentrate on the next assessment (of which there are many) to pass. However, all of the activities were delivered in schools with a high proportion of pupils from an educationally and socially disadvantaged background and were designed to be sustainable learning and teaching resources for the schools and for our WP outreach. A good number of resources are still run through our Peninsula Pathways to Medicine outreach through our WAMS ambassadors. However, WAMS is an independent society whose chair and committee change every year. The inevitable lack of continuity meant that they were not always willing or had time to take up some of the many extra resources and lesson plans that were produced through this module. Teddy Bear Hospital stations with activities designed in the SSU are still run in many primary schools as well as a poster and lesson plan to teach Year 6 pupils Basic Life Support Skills, which was a feature at a yearly three-week-long event for pupils transitioning to secondary schools called Junior Life Skills.

Our Widening Access to Medicine students also utilise an SSU resource to familiarise aspiring medical students with the multi-mini-interviews used for selection to medical school.

The SSU resources used by our own student outreach team in the primary and secondary schools are featured in the case studies (Box 1).

Unintended consequences/impact

This project had many unintended consequences including the success of a pilot study and the continuation of the widening participation projects in the Doctors as Educators module to this day. The module has evolved over the years due to changes in the SSU structure and an increased number of medical students following a government directive.

The longevity of some of the resources was not intended. A great example are the stations designed for our Teddy Bear Hospitals to primary school children (Box 1). Many of the activities were designed as part of Doctors as Educators and are still delivered to this day in our primary schools in the most deprived parts of Plymouth. These sessions deliver health-related messages alongside aspirational aspects, which aim to plant the seed of medicine as a potential career. These sessions have been taken up by local charities in Plymouth who work with the most deprived children in the city.

Some of the resources were adapted to different settings, for example, to a 'short station structure' and became important contributions to larger scale interventions. One such resource, designed by a 4th Year student to teach children basic life support also became a feature of an annual 'Junior Life Skills' event for Year 6 school pupils. The original lesson plan and Dr ABC poster were adapted for a face-to-face hands-on session. Through Junior Life Skills, this project taught basic life skills to thousands of children and accompanied school staff for many years. In total, 3,700 Year 6 pupils from 54 schools engaged each year with this key learning during the Junior Life Skills event. Another unintended but remarkable consequence resulted in a teacher expressing immense gratitude a year later. This teacher used basic life skills successfully to save her husband whilst they waited for an ambulance. The Junior Life Skills is no longer running but WAMS have adapted the resource and lesson plan to deliver the same sessions in local schools.

Our WAMS students also deliver resources designed in the Doctors as Educators SSU to familiarise aspiring medical students with the Multi-Mini-Medical Selection Interviews used in many medical schools as a key selection tool. The sessions relayed key information about medical selection followed by a 'mock' MMI for all the school students.

A few medical students from traditionally privileged backgrounds who took up this SSU were able to interact and engage with young children from a very different demographic. The students gained an insight into not only communicating and engaging with children but also understanding some of the issues related to the social determinants of health and real-life illustrations that they may not have been previously aware of. These interactions will be invaluable in their future as a doctor. Furthermore, many of the medical students developed a deeper understanding and increased awareness of the reasons behind the National drive to Widening Participation in medicine and the health and social issues for some children in Plymouth whether they took up a school/WP project or not.

Finally, some resources went further afield. Students took activities and resources to schools near their homes. An example includes medical students who delivered sessions including multi-mini-interview, surgery skills, and reflection in schools close to home in East London.

Conclusion

In conclusion, the Widening Access/Student Selected Unit projects brought health education in schools to life via the direct input of medical students. It was a welcome and exciting addition for the schools – especially in the light of increasing budgetary constraints and changing PSHEE to non-statutory status on both devolved funding to all schools as well as that allocated to the Local Authority. It allowed schools to address a wide variety of topics within the PSHEE framework. Importantly, it also made a career in health a more accessible concept to children and young people by bringing them into direct contact with medical students from a similar background to themselves.

Medical students learned the theory and practice of teaching and learning, and gained experience in engaging and communicating with a wide demographic of people from different ages, and socio-economic groups. They learned to adapt their communication skills appropriately and also gained valuable experience in health education and practical insights into the social determinants of health.

Finally, our WP strategy became more focused and targeted through strong connections with the Education Directorate at Plymouth City Council. We gained local knowledge and thus access to local children from the most deprived areas and under-represented demographic at university and in particular Medicine. Finally, we gained and continue to gain innovative, novel, sustainable resources and lesson plans each year from these talented students.

References

BBC. (2023). *BBC Report on Sex Education Review*. www.bbc.co.uk/news/uk-politics-64892868

Françoise Granoulhac. (2018). Making schools work for the economy: Education discourse and policies from David Cameron to Theresa May. https://journals.openedition.org/osb/2322

GMC Outcomes for Graduate. (2020). www.gmc-uk.org/education/standards-guidance-and-curricula/standards-and-outcomes/outcomes-for-graduates/outcomes-for-graduates

Medical Schools Council. (2014). *Selecting for Excellence Report.* www.medschools.ac.uk/media/1203/selecting-for-excellence-final-report.pdf

Milburn, A. (2012). Fair access to professional careers. *The Independent Reviewer on Social Mobility and Child Poverty.* https://assets.publishing.service.gov.uk/media/5a78a420e5274a277e68e514/IR_FairAccess_acc2.pdf

Ofsted Handbook. (2022). *Personal Development Guidance about Teaching Personal, Social, Health and Economic (PSHE) Education in England.*

Plymouth City Council. (2012). www.plymouth.gov.uk/sites/default/files/media-uploads/Child_poverty_needs_assessment_2012.pdf

Stone, G. (2017). www.sec-ed.co.uk/content/best-practice/curriculum-the-influence-of-ed-hirsch/

Sutton Trust. (2019). *Elitist Britain 2019.* www.suttontrust.com/wp-content/uploads/2020/01/Elitist-Britain-2019-Summary-Report.pdf

UK Government. (2013). *Guidance about Teaching Personal, Social, Health and Economic (PSHE) Education in England.* www.gov.uk/government/publications/personal-social-health-and-economic-education-pshe

Chapter 4

Encouraging student research and engagement in widening participation

Enam Haque, Ben Ryan, Robert Cartwright-Speakman, Nadin Hawwash, Danielle Nimmons, and Umair Gondal

Importance of student involvement in WP research and engagement

There are different ways that medical students can get involved in WP research and engagement. The first case study looks at the 'Widening Participation Fellow' Programme in Manchester, whereby medical students doing intercalated research master's degrees can apply for a one-year role as a WP fellow. The tasks of this role include designing, delivering, and evaluating student engagement activities from primary to secondary schools, and also providing the student voice on the WP Committee in medical school.

Students have used their medical studies as well as their free time to engage in outreach activities and research on their work. The next three cases focus on examples of projects that have had marked input. The first case outlines the work of Manchester Outreach Medics (MOMs), a student society that runs widening access initiatives in Greater Manchester and Lancashire. MOMs have successfully published their work, and the case study highlights some of their projects. The second case covers a project undertaken by a Year 3 medical student, as part of a project module in the MB ChB programme. They developed an outreach event in a 'cold spot' area, where few pupils went into higher education. Their work is outlined, utilising literature to create a validated intervention for Year 9 pupils. The final case is a virtual online resource for school pupils to use, to get an idea about medicine as a career. This asynchronous offering was developed by an intercalating MB-PhD medical student, during their time as a WP Fellow. The idea was conceived, delivered, and evaluated by them. The chapter concludes with a discussion on the merits of different evaluation methods that demonstrate impact for students, and implications for their future career development.

Case Study 1: WP fellow programme – Dr Danielle Nimmons and Dr Umair Gondal

The University of Manchester's Widening Participation Fellow Programme allows students studying a higher degree in any discipline to plan, lead, and

DOI: 10.4324/9781003399858-4

deliver a range of educational activities for school pupils aged 10–18 years, with the aim to attract talented school pupils from under-represented groups onto university courses. From 2011, up to four medical students undertaking master's degrees during intercalated years can join the programme, whose main focus is on STEM subjects and in particular, access into medicine.

The scheme is a period of paid employment over ten months, including 100 hours of work that are logged, including the planning and evaluation of activities, not only the delivery. Students are required to be WP Ambassadors for their Faculty and School, linking in with other staff, students, young people, and community groups. It is also an opportunity to network and collaborate with other WP Fellows and academic staff in the delivery of activities, and to raise awareness of WP.

Training is provided at the start of the year and over a period of weeks. This provides a foundation for teaching skills, including the planning of engaging activities and providing feedback to a range of learners from different backgrounds. There is a wide breadth of activities covered, tailored to different age groups, and can include, for example, science workshops and career events. All activities are formally evaluated, which is used to strengthen the WP activities of subsequent years.

WP fellow perspectives

DANIELLE: WP FELLOW FROM 2012 TO 2013

'The Fellow Programme provided a strong foundation for my subsequent teaching and academic career to date. Before any teaching activities took place there were around 10 hours of protected paid time for training, which included how to plan teaching for different learners and age groups and how to obtain useful feedback. This ensured we had the necessary skills to deliver effective and impactful teaching.

There was a great choice of teaching activities available to take part in on our own or in pairs. For example, I developed an open day for school students interested in studying medicine with another WP Fellow and hosted a session on my own titled 'Medicine Through the Ages' at the Manchester Museum, using their artefacts and objects as part of the session. Feedback from schoolteachers and students was positive and knowing I had inspired students from underrepresented groups to pursue medicine was incredibly rewarding.

I also taught in schools and colleges about my research at the time, which was on swallowing problems in older people. This was the first time I was able to appreciate the link between teaching and research, which opened my eyes to the possibility of a clinical academic career. Since being a WP Fellow,

I have developed my academic skills further and am currently conducting a PhD which includes health inequalities in dementia, and this research informs my teaching.'

Further reflections on her experience as a WP Fellow can be found at Azmy and Nimmons (2017).

UMAIR: WP FELLOW FROM 2015 TO 2016

'As a Widening Participation Fellow, I was able to organise workshops that brought science to life for high school students. One memorable event involved developing a session that allowed students to create a game to understand gas exchange in the lungs. This hands-on experience not only kindled their curiosity but also offered insights into how science translates into the medical field. What made this experience particularly rewarding was the opportunity it provided for students from less privileged backgrounds to interact with medical students, breaking down barriers and fostering an inclusive educational environment. As someone who attended these low-participating schools myself, I found it particularly enjoyable to provide support to students who may have the academic ability but not the opportunities to progress into higher education. The positive feedback I received from these initiatives was a testament to their impact.

Yet, my journey as a WP Fellow extended beyond the tangible benefits to the students. It was a personal transformation. The role demanded time management, bolstered my confidence, and honed my organisational skills. These qualities have proven invaluable in my career as a doctor. Whether it's navigating a hectic hospital schedule or confidently addressing patients' concerns, the experiences as a WP Fellow continue to serve as a foundation for my professional growth.'

Benefits and challenges

The role of a Widening Participation Fellow is both rewarding and challenging, providing valuable experiences and opportunities for personal and professional growth. WP Fellows play a vital role in fostering connections between young learners and higher education. This role is not without its challenges, as it demands effective time management to balance academic commitments with outreach responsibilities. Additionally, WP Fellows often face the task of finding the right balance between their various responsibilities, which can be demanding.

Moreover, coordinating events and building connections with local schools and communities can be resource-intensive, requiring meticulous planning and substantial networking efforts. It is also essential to establish clear selection criteria to target students and schools with the greatest need.

However, the benefits of the role are profound. WP Fellows acquire essential skills such as time management, leadership, and organisation, which are valuable in various professional contexts. Financial support often accompanies the role, and the opportunity to network with university staff helps Fellows develop as role models for their communities and subject areas.

The impact of the programme extends to attendees, as they receive support for their future and career development, and a boost in their aspirations. The programme also increases their association with the local university, allowing them to gain insights into university life from current students. In a broader context, the university benefits by using the programme as a recruitment tool for prospective students, all while solidifying its commitment to supporting the local community.

Tips for universities who want to implement WP fellows

Robust Selection Criteria: Establish clear and focused selection criteria, targeting WP students and schools with low progression rates into university, particularly in lower socio-economic locations.

Record Hours: Ensure rigorous logging of hours to justify payment and monitor WP Fellow work effectively.

Feedback Loop: Emphasis on the importance of feedback from schools and students to fine-tune the programme and improve its effectiveness. Feedback can also be used as evidence of teaching for the Fellows' CV.

Institutional Buy-In: Secure the support and buy-in of the university to ensure that the programme is integrated successfully into the institution's educational outreach efforts.

Community Engagement: Develop and maintain strong relationships with local schools and colleges to facilitate the collaboration and outreach needed to make the programme a success.

Comprehensive Training: Invest in the training of Fellows, providing them with essential skills such as lesson plan development. We advise ensuring there is protected (and paid) time for this.

Case Study 2: Manchester Outreach Medics (MOMs) – Dr Ben Ryan and Dr Enam Haque

Manchester Outreach Medics is a medical student-led society that runs events for Year 12 pupils with WP flags in the Lancashire and Greater Manchester area. It was founded in 2015 and is supported by the University of Manchester and local hospital NHS trusts. The events are free to attend and aim to empower attendees. This is by supporting them with the application process to medical school and by providing insight into life as a medical student and doctor. The project leaders received guidance on delivering events from staff in the WP team at UoM Medical School. This improved their evaluation methods and led to the design of a simple and feasible means of assessing the efficacy of their events. These were pre- and post-intervention questionnaires which attendees completed, highlighting their understanding in different areas on a zero to ten scale. These evaluation methods were key for the project leader to identify areas for improvement and led to the publication of a research article about their events (Ryan et al., 2018). This collaborative working with the medical school enabled the MOMs team to grow in terms of their personal and professional development, consistent with Vygotsky's Zone of Proximal Development (Vygotsky, 1978) and encouraged further engagement.

One component of the Manchester MB ChB curriculum is a Year 3 student-selected project, called the Applied Personal Excellence Pathway (APEP), during which students conduct literature reviews and their own research. The author used this academic opportunity to design, develop, and evaluate a bespoke event for Year 12 pupils. A review of the literature highlighted that pupils from disadvantaged areas were less likely to apply to medicine as they lacked confidence in their abilities (Mathers and Perry, 2009; McHarg et al., 2007). To address this, he designed a unique intervention: a conference for sixth form pupils to attend and deliver their own presentations. Pupils were supported by the author to research a topic of their choosing and create a brief presentation on it. At the conference, pupils delivered their presentations to a group of their peers and a panel of medical student volunteers. Pre- and post-intervention questionnaires asked pupils to highlight their confidence in different areas on a scale of zero to ten. The data demonstrated a significant improvement in confidence, with a large effect size in most areas assessed (Ryan et al., 2021). The author achieved a distinction grade in the summative assessment of the APEP, demonstrating the academic rigour with which the WP project was undertaken. This could be explained by the added motivation to engage in active learning, as the author was pursuing their interest in developing a WP initiative. The success of the conference led to it being added as an annual event by MOMs. The research element of the conference was also adapted by the author for his innovative access programme, Lancashire Access Medics (LAM). This is covered in a later chapter by the same author (Chapter 8). Year 12 pupils taking part in LAM complete a research project over the summer and deliver a presentation to a panel of junior doctor volunteers. This case study highlights the benefits of medical schools incorporating socially responsible academic projects into their curricula. It provides the opportunity for students to engage in non-traditional but important work. By doing so, students may be more engaged in their work, improving their motivation to learn, and developing additional skills to develop a portfolio in WP outreach.

Case Study 3: Widening participation in Wigan – Dr Robert Cartwright-Speakman and Dr Enam Haque

The MSC Selection Alliance identified cold spot areas that required more efforts to widen access into medicine (MSC, 2019). Cold spots are defined as areas that have little to no outreach initiatives for students wanting to apply to medical school (MSC, 2020). One such cold-spot area was Wigan, a working-class town located in the north-west of England in which there was not a culture of applying to higher education. 31.1% of children from Wigan lived in poverty and less than 50% of pupils left secondary school with a grade C or above in English and Math (GM Poverty Action, 2022; UK Gov, 2023). The author of this chapter was born and bred there. He was the only pupil from his school year who successfully applied to Medicine and was the first member of his family to go to university. As a medical student, he wanted to improve the opportunities for pupils in his hometown, to raise their aspirations and improve their awareness of Medicine as a career. He formulated a bespoke widening participation initiative during his MB ChB studies, as part of his third-year project module. This was one of the first projects to look at widening participation as part of an academic exercise. It aimed to evaluate the impact of an intervention to challenge perceived barriers that high school pupils had to studying medicine. This intervention consisted of a workshop that informed pupils on the barriers to applying to medicine, as well as ways to overcome these.

Key barriers to studying medicine include

1   Parental attitudes towards higher education
2   Personal attitude towards perceived academic ability
3   Lack of knowledge towards application to medicine
4   Peer attitudes towards higher education
5   Financial attitude towards the cost of university

These identified barriers (Callender and Jackson, 2005; Grbic et al., 2015; Hill et al., 2004; Maras, 2007; Martin et al., 2018) were embedded in the design of the workshop, creating solutions to address each of them as far as possible.

Recruitment

Schools in Wigan were chosen based on Attainment 8 scores, reflecting pupils' achievement in up to eight qualifications (UK Gov, 2019; AQA, 2019). They were contacted via an email which outlined the aims of the workshop. One school with a below-average Attainment 8 score was recruited for the study. The pupils selected to take part were in Y9 and had high grades and Cognitive Ability Test (CAT) scores. CAT scores were selected as these are indicative of GCSE performance (GL Assessment, 2019).

Workshop design

The workshop consisted of an interactive presentation tackling these five barriers. The author incorporated his own experiences of these barriers into the workshop, as well as highlighting how he addressed them. Addressing the barrier of negative parental attitudes, the author emphasised to pupils that they should discuss their ideas for higher education with their parents. He shared how he informed his parents of how the medicine application process worked. By including them, he was able to receive support from them when applying to medical schools. In terms of low academic self-esteem, he narrated his story of being dissuaded by teachers from taking triple science as it would '*distract other students who want to be doctors*'. He highlighted the irony of this statement and the importance of pupils believing in themselves. He advised pupils to brush off negative comments from teachers. In terms of knowledge of the medicine application, the author asked pupils to tell him their hobbies and voluntary activities. He then asked them what skills they felt a doctor needed, and whether their hobbies and voluntary work mapped to these skills. He explained the application process and key activities to successfully steer through this. In terms of lack of peer support, the author highlighted the importance of being surrounded by like-minded individuals and stressed the benefits of having long-term goals over short-term benefits. He addressed the financial barrier by highlighting the job security medicine presented as well as providing information on student loans and how they were paid off. The session ended with a teaching session on chest X-ray interpretation. This enabled students to believe they could perform like a doctor, to motivate them to learn more about a career in medicine.

Evaluation

The author evaluated the impact of the workshop with a paper Likert scale questionnaire exploring pupil perception of the five barriers to Medicine. The questionnaire was distributed randomly to all participants. Pupils signed a written consent to use the results of the workshop in research, at the start of the paper questionnaire. They then completed the questionnaire before and after the intervention. Each questionnaire had a distinct number so that the pre-workshop and post-workshop questionnaires could be paired for each pupil.

Ethics

The University of Manchester Ethics Decision Tool was used to assess the need for ethics approval, given participants were under 18 years old. No ethics application was deemed necessary as all information collated was anonymous and did not collect any personally identifiable data.

Analysis

To determine significance, separate paired t-tests were conducted for self-attitudes and resource knowledge data. Three Wilcoxon tests evaluated the data for the remaining barriers. The respective tests for each barrier were selected based on their Shapiro–Wilk score.

Results

100% of the students thought that the workshop was useful and 96% stated they would like to take part in similar future workshops. Attitudes towards knowledge of resources, finances, self-belief, and parental support significantly improved (p <0.01) with the intervention.

Learning from the workshop

This innovative student-led workshop demonstrated a positive impact on pupils who attended. It also showed how medical students could utilise their academic projects to make positive change in widening participation. It was positively received as a presentation at the National Medical

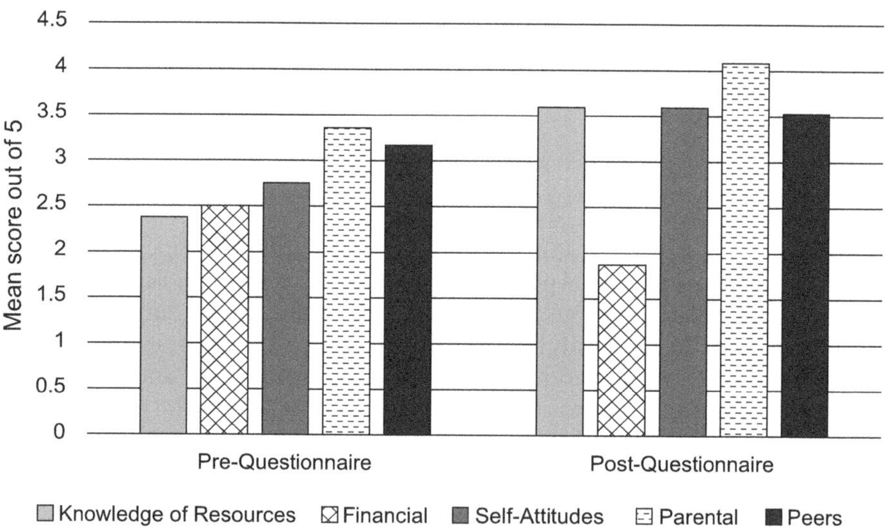

Figure 4.1 A graph showing the mean difference in attitudes towards barriers to medicine before and after engagement in the presentation

Source: The only barrier that did not produce a statistically significant improvement was pupil perception of the importance of having good peer support. This may have been due to them not considering the importance of peers before the workshop and needed time to consider this

Schools Widening Participation Forum's Annual National Conference in 2019. The plan is now to develop the workshop into a sustainable outreach programme.

Case Study 4: Plant a seed series: a case study on the impact of an online outreach package on school pupils' knowledge, skills, and attitudes to medicine – Dr Nadin Hawwash and Dr Enam Haque

Medicine is one of the most inaccessible professions for social mobility (1). Widening participation (WP) initiatives in the United Kingdom (UK) have primarily focused on either pupils attending primary school or in Years 10 to 13. However, as seen in the outreach work in Wigan, the critical age for raising awareness of a career in medicine is Years 7–9. Pupils are then able to consider GCSE subjects and grade requirements for studying medicine before they finalise their courses.

The project

The previous case study looked at an in-person outreach activity. This case looks at the innovative use of asynchronous, online video resources to break down barriers to medicine. In 2022, the authors created a national initiative, titled the Plant a Seed (PAS) series. This was an online pre-recorded series uploaded on the University of Manchester website, to 'Inspire', 'Educate', and 'Motivate' pupils from WP backgrounds into medicine. The PAS series consisted of three sessions lasting between 30 and 60 minutes and each began with a short clip of the day in the life of a doctor. The 'Inspire' session focused on the history of heart surgery and the development of vaccines. The 'Educate' session focused on the anatomy of the lungs, pathophysiology, diagnosis, and treatment of asthma. The 'Motivate' session focused on the journey of a medical student through higher education. The team explored the impact of PAS on pupils' knowledge, skills, and attitude to Medicine and medical applications. This was through a national pretest–posttest study of pupils in participating secondary schools in the United Kingdom (UK). Following ethics approval, the Higher Education Access Tracker (HEAT) was used to compile a list of 500 UK secondary schools in widening participation postcodes. All schools on the list were invited to take part in PAS. Seventy pupils in Years 7–9 from two schools participated in this study. Consented pupils viewed all three episodes of PAS and completed a pre- and post-series online questionnaire. A Likert scale measured pupil confidence in terms of knowledge, skills, and attitudes towards a medical career. The series demonstrated a significant increase in pupil knowledge of the role and life of a doctor, what a medical degree entailed, admissions requirements, and future careers in medicine (p <0.05). There was a significant increase in pupils believing they could apply to and study medicine. However, there was an insignificant increase in pupils wanting to study medicine after the series (p = 0.187).

Implications

The PAS series significantly improved the knowledge, skills, and confidence of pupils, demonstrating the benefit to enrolment of the programme at scale. However, the course did not significantly increase the number of pupils wishing to study medicine. A contributing factor to the small sample size and number of schools enrolled onto the series included the limited duration of advertisement of PAS, given significant delays with ethics approval. Additionally, each school participating in the series was required to commit to viewing three 30–60-minute videos over the course of the academic year. Despite the opportunity to watch the series at any suitable time, a level of long-term commitment from each school was required. As a research study, the PAS series study also required some level of administrative support with the requirement to distribute and collect (i) an assent form, (ii) participant information sheet, (iii) parent consent form, (iv) PAS worksheet, and (v) a certificate of attendance which may have discouraged schools enrolling onto the series.

Reflections

Virtual widening participation strategies conducted as a series of sessions have proven to be effective in increasing pupils' understanding of medicine. Distribution of PAS via schools was necessary to ensure technological accessibility; however, this format of distribution and exposure to PAS was highly dependent on each school's commitment. Analysis at scale with a duration of advertisement, enrolment, and follow-up is required to evaluate the effectiveness of the PAS series as a key intervention to break down barriers to medicine.

Evaluation

As seen in the case studies, students have utilised pre- and post-session evaluation questionnaires to demonstrate the impact of their intervention. This quantitative measure enables statistical analysis to be performed, to demonstrate significant change. However, there are two aspects that this approach does not measure. The first is longitudinal and lasting benefit of the intervention. Secondly, the qualitative perspective, to gain a deeper understanding of the impact of the intervention. Plant a Seed tries to address the limitations of a standalone intervention, offering a series of video resources, for school pupils to access over a period of time. However, again this evaluated the series from a largely quantitative perspective.

Moving forward, students should consider mixed methods studies, utilising quantitative and qualitative methods. They should ensure ethics approval is sought, particularly for the qualitative approach. The study could include focus groups or individual interviews, to gauge a deeper understanding of the impact of an intervention. Interventions need to move away from standalone activities to a series of activities, which help pupils grow in their knowledge, skills, and attitude towards a career in medicine.

The main barrier to making this a reality is the limited time that medical students and academics have for designing, delivering, and evaluating their interventions. Faculty needs to consider WP as a key area of research, and to enable students and academics the time and space to develop their academic interest.

References

AQA. (2019). *Attainment 8*. www.aqa.org.uk/about-us/what-we-do/policy/gcse-and-a-level-changes/attainment-8

Azmy, J., and Nimmons, D. (2017, April). Reflections on a widening participation teaching role. *Clinical Teacher*, 14(2), 139–140.

Baker, H., and Sela, K. (2018). The role of the student ambassador and its contribution to developing employability skills: A creation of outward facing work roles. In: D. Morley (ed.), *Enhancing Employability in Higher Education through Work Based Learning*. Cham: Palgrave Macmillan. https://doi.org/10.1007/978-3-319-75166-5_11

Callender, C., and Jackson, J. (2005). Does the fear of debt deter students from higher education? *Journal of Social Policy*, 34(4), 509–540.

GL Assessment. (2019). www.gl-assessment.co.uk/sites/gl/files/images/Files/GCSE_Technical_Information.pdf

GM Poverty Action. (2022). www.gmpovertyaction.org/pm2022-child-poverty/ (accessed 24 July 2023)

Grbic, D., Jones, D. J., and Case, S. T. (2015). The role of socioeconomic status in medical school admissions: Validation of a socioeconomic indicator for use in medical school admissions. *Academic Medicine*, 90(7), 953–960.

Haque, E., Kardasz, A., and Alldridge, L. (2021). What impact does teaching in outreach activities have on medical students' own learning and teaching skills? A pilot study. *Widening Participation and Lifelong Learning*, 23(2), 20, 152–163(12).

Hill, N. E., Castellino, D. R., Lansford, J. E., Nowlin, P., Dodge, K. A., Bates, J. E., and Pettit, G. S. (2004). Parent academic involvement as related to school behavior, achievement, and aspirations: Demographic variations across adolescence. *Child Development*, 75(5), 1491–1509.

Maras, P. (2007). "But no one in my family has been to university" aiming higher: School students' attitudes to higher education. *The Australian Educational Researcher*, 34(3), 69–90.

Martin, A. J., Beska, B. J., Wood, G., Wyatt, N., Codd, A., Vance, G., and Burford, B. (2018). Widening interest, widening participation: Factors influencing school students' aspirations to study medicine. *BMC Medical Education*, 18(1), 117.

Mathers, J., and Parry, J. (2009). Why are there so few working-class applicants to medical schools? Learning from the success stories. *Medical Education*, 43(3), 219–228. doi: 10.1111/j.1365-2923.2008.03274.x

McHarg, J., Mattick, K., and Knight, L. V. (2007). Why people apply to medical school: Implications for widening participation activities. *Medical Education*, 41(8), 815–821. doi: 10.1111/j.1365-2923

MSC. (2019). www.medschools.ac.uk/media/2608/selection-alliance-2019-report.pdf

MSC.(2020).www.medschools.ac.uk/media/2806/msc-summer-schools-annual-report.pdf (accessed 31 July 2023)

Ryan, B., Auty, C., Maden, M., Leggett, A., Staley, A., and Haque, E. (2021). Widening participation in medicine: The impact of medical student-led conferences for year 12 pupils. *Advances in Medical Education Practice*, 12, 937–943. doi: 10.2147/AMEP.S314581

Ryan, B., Kitchen, A., Chan, A., Gibson, H., and Haque, E. (2018). Widening participation to medicine: A student-led workshop for medical school applicants. *MedEdPublish*, 7, 130. doi: 10.15694/mep.2018.0000130.1

UK GOV. (2019). www.compare-school-performance.service.gov.uk/compare-schools?for=secondary&orderby=ks4.0.P8_BANDING&orderdir=asc

UKGOV.(2023).www.find-school-performance-data.service.gov.uk/school/106534/the-deanery-church-of-england-high-school-and-sixth-form-college/secondary

Vygotsky, L. S. (1978). *Mind in Society: Development of Higher Psychological Processes* (M. Cole, V. Jolm-Steiner, S. Scribner, and E. Souberman, eds.). Harvard University Press. doi: 10.2307/j.ctvjf9vz4

Chapter 5

Career-focused outreach – Medicine Calling

A case study

Samuel Adcock, Sarah Kasher, and Rachel Winter

Introduction and background

Psychiatry has struggled to recruit and retain sufficient doctors for some time (Mukherjee et al., 2013; Henfrey, 2015; Shields et al., 2017) at a time when demand for psychiatric services continually increases (Royal College of Psychiatrists, 2020). The factors that have affected recruitment to psychiatry historically are multiple, complex, and not fully understood. A negative, inaccurate, and stigmatised view of psychiatry and psychiatric patients is not uncommon among medical students or doctors (Balon et al., 1999; Laugharne et al., 2009; Dixon et al., 2008; Lyons, 2013). Knowledge amongst medical students about psychiatry as a profession remains limited (Deb and Lomax, 2014), and much of what is believed about psychiatry presents it as outdated, inaccurate, unscientific, and unrewarding (Mukherjee et al., 2013; Deb and Lomax, 2014). Issues with recruitment to mental health services are not just limited to psychiatry. Around 12% of all medical vacancies are in mental health services (BMA, 2020), with mental health nursing vacancies accounting for nearly a third of all unfilled nurse posts across England (Palmer et al., 2023).

These issues with recruitment, alongside the publication of the NHS Long Term Workforce Plan in 2023 (NHS, 2023), which has several ambitious targets, including growing the number of staff working in the mental health sector, demonstrate more than ever the importance of attracting increasing numbers of young people into mental health careers. However, Medicine Calling has found young people aspire to work in the sector, but they do not fully understand the different career options. For example, 139 Year 12 students who attended a Medicine Calling event during 2020–2021 were asked, 'Prior to attending Medicine Calling, did you know the difference between a psychiatrist and a psychologist?' 53% of students answered 'No' to this question. A recent paper evaluating the knowledge of and attitudes relating to psychiatry and clinical psychology in A-level students also reported knowledge was generally poor with only 57% of respondents knowing that psychiatrists had medical degrees (Morgan et al., 2021). These findings highlight the confusion amongst young people surrounding different professions in the sector.

DOI: 10.4324/9781003399858-5

Further research was carried out by Medicine Calling in early 2020, where the team conducted focus groups in three schools in Leicestershire with Year 12 students who had an interest in studying psychology at university. Results found that the majority of participants had never heard of psychiatry or were unsure of what the role entailed, despite many participants expressing a desire to support and work with people suffering from a mental illness in the future. Most participants had never considered alternatives to psychology such as mental health nursing. Responses from focus group participants included:

"I thought it was all one, I assumed a psychiatrist was the same as a psychologist."

"I spoke to our careers advisor, and she spoke a lot about psychologists but never really mentioned a psychiatrist."

"I thought psychiatrist was an American term, whereas we would call them psychologists."

These findings further identify the misconceptions around mental health careers among young people and the importance of providing education and information around careers in mental health to school and college students.

Several publications have also highlighted the disparity across schools and colleges with regard to careers information provided to young people. Research shows students who are eligible for free school meals or attend a school or college in a deprived area of England are less likely to have access to a specialist careers adviser or service (White et al., 2022; House of Commons Education Committee, 2023). As a result, Medicine Calling focuses on working with schools and colleges that have a high proportion of students who meet various widening participation indicators. Typically, this includes schools and colleges with a high proportion of students who live in an area of deprivation or low progression onto higher education; students who live or have experience of local authority care; or students who have claimed free school meals in the last six years. Thus, helping to ensure that all students are able to access accurate workforce information. In addition, Medicine Calling believes working with students from a range of different backgrounds is essential to attract a diverse future mental health workforce that is representative of the communities they serve.

Combined, these findings demonstrate the importance of career-focused outreach programmes, such as Medicine Calling, for school and college students. They aim to ensure young people not only have the correct information but access to resources to allow them to make an informed decision about their future career. This is arguably even more important with medicine and healthcare professions, as the majority of university courses in these fields require prospective applicants to meet increasingly specific entry requirements.

Medicine Calling's main aims are to

- Increase students' understanding of psychiatry and what a psychiatrist does.
- Increase the number of students considering becoming a psychiatrist or mental health nurse in the future.
- Increase students' awareness of the range of careers connected to mental health.

In order to meet Medicine Calling's aims, all activity is designed to meet the following objectives:

- To provide a welcoming environment for students to learn about psychiatry, mental health nursing, and other professions in mental health.
- To delineate psychiatry from other associated disciplines, for example, psychology, explaining the similarities and differences.
- To equip students with knowledge about careers in medicine, so they understand what psychiatry entails in comparison to other medical and surgical disciplines.
- To raise awareness about the opportunities a career in psychiatry can offer, including various subspecialties.
- To challenge and dispel some of the negative, inaccurate, and stigmatised views of psychiatry and mental health that are prevalent both within the general public and medical profession.
- To offer students an insight into life as a medical and nursing student, junior doctor, trainee, and consultant psychiatrist and mental health nurse with the opportunity to take part in practical workshops.
- To provide students with the knowledge of the different routes into working in mental health with emphasis on routes into becoming a psychiatrist and mental health nurse.
- To inspire students to consider a career in psychiatry and mental health nursing by allowing them to meet and hear from doctors and nurses who are both passionate about the discipline and proud to work in the sector.

Results

To achieve these aims and objectives, since 2016, Medicine Calling has organised several large-scale conferences and careers evenings for students in Years 7 to 13. These events provide a platform for students to find out more about different careers in the mental health sector. Students from across the UK, with a focus on those residing in the Midlands, are invited to the University of Leicester, where they can attend a variety of talks and workshops. These showcase different mental health professions and attendees can meet current students and healthcare professionals (see Appendix 1 for an example programme). At all events, attendees are also informed about the skills and qualifications they need in order to pursue these careers. During 2020–2022, several events were adapted and delivered online due to Covid restrictions.

Since 2022, Medicine Calling has continued to offer online sessions alongside face-to-face events to provide an alternative for students who may find it difficult to travel to the University of Leicester.

Each year, Medicine Calling organises specific events to target different age groups. For example, a Year 12 and 13 Medicine Calling Conference; a Year 10 and 11 Medicine Calling Careers Evening; and a Year 7, 8, and 9 Medicine Calling Taster Day. At each event, the format and content are adapted in order to be appropriate and relevant to the age group. The approach to recruiting students to each event is adapted as needed. For example, with the Year 7, 8, and 9 Medicine Calling Taster Day, local schools and colleges with a high proportion of widening participation students are invited to bring a group of students to the event. Medicine Calling asks schools and colleges to select a group of students, with at least 50% who meet a minimum of one widening participation criterion, as well as students who have an interest or the potential to pursue a career in healthcare. This exposes a diverse group of students, who may never have considered a career in mental health, to the possibility of a career in the sector.

Medicine Calling believes working with younger students is essential if more are going to be attracted to work in mental health, as evidence suggests young people only consider careers that are familiar to them (House of Commons Education Committee, 2023). However, the Sutton Trust recently reported only 5% of Year 7 students had attended an employer talk or event (White et al., 2022) demonstrating how younger year groups often miss out on career-led outreach and opportunities. As a result, younger students are a key audience for Medicine Calling.

Impact

All students apply to attend a Medicine Calling event through HEAT, an online tracking and monitoring database used by the University of Leicester. As part of the HEAT form, students or their parents/carers are asked to provide their postcode, gender, and ethnicity, as well as answer questions about free school meal eligibility. This allows simple and reliable analysis of the demographic information of attendees and ensures Medicine Calling is working with students from a range of different backgrounds. Medicine Calling also asks all attendees to complete a pre-event questionnaire to help understand what students already know, as well as an end-of-event evaluation form to analyse the impact of the event.

Project aim: Increase students' understanding of psychiatry and what a psychiatrist does

Since 2016, in the post-event evaluation form, 100% of attendees stated that they felt more knowledgeable about psychiatry as a profession after attending a Medicine Calling event, which is fantastic and demonstrates how Medicine Calling is raising awareness of psychiatry among young people.

Project aim 1: Increase the number of students considering becoming a psychiatrist or mental health nurse in the future

All attendees are asked in both the pre-event questionnaire and end-of-event evaluation form if they are considering a career in psychiatry. As *Figure 5.1* demonstrates, there is a significant increase in the number of students who, after attending a Medicine Calling event, would now consider becoming a psychiatrist in the future, which is extremely positive.

As Medicine Calling also hopes to inspire students into wider careers within the mental health sector, at more recent events, students were also asked whether or not they are considering a career in mental health generally. As *Figure 5.2* demonstrates, there was a significant increase in the number of students considering a career in the mental health sector after attending a Medicine Calling event, suggesting the event portrayed a range of careers in the sector positively. If students answered 'Yes' to this question, they were asked what careers they were considering. Responses included psychiatrist, mental health nurse, general practitioner, psychologist, and therapist. It is also worth highlighting the significant increase in the number of students considering a career in the sector after the March 2023 event. This event targeted students in Years 7, 8, and 9, which further supports the importance of working with younger students to help raise awareness of careers they may be unfamiliar with.

Project aim 2: Increase students' awareness of the range of careers connected to mental illness

Students are asked in both the pre-event questionnaire and end-of-event evaluation to rate their knowledge on a range of topics on a scale of 1–5, with 1

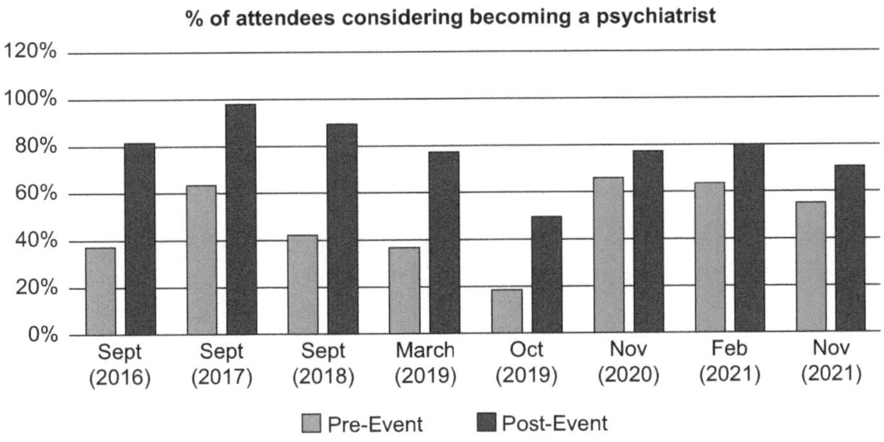

Figure 5.1 Graph to illustrate changes in opinions regarding psychiatry as a career pre- and post-intervention

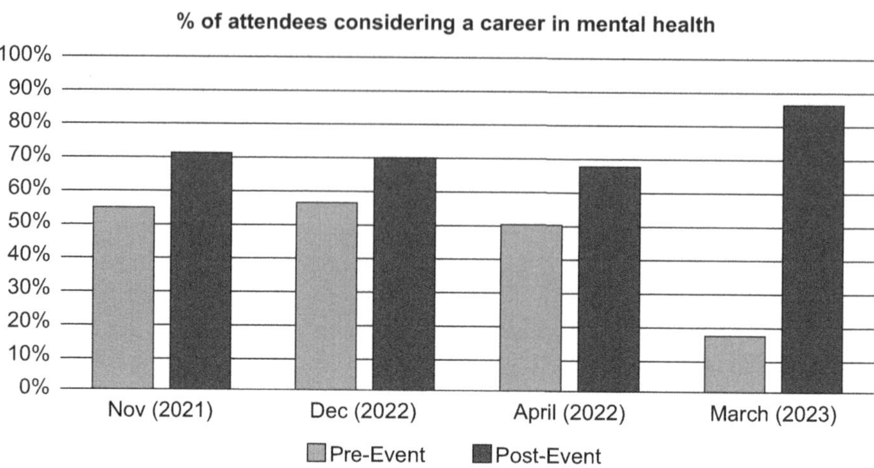

Figure 5.2 Graph to illustrate changes in opinions regarding a career in mental health pre- and post-intervention

being not confident at all and 5 being extremely confident. *Figure 5.3* presents the results of students who attended an event during 2021–2023. When asked about their knowledge of different careers in the mental health sector, students said they felt more knowledgeable about the range of careers in mental health after attending an event, fulfilling this particular project's aim.

Anecdotal feedback from Medicine Calling events has also been extremely positive and further demonstrates how the events are helping to inform students about the range of careers in the mental health sector:

- I now understand what psychiatrists and psychologists do and how I could potentially pursue a career in that field. I especially liked how interactive the event was and the fact that all my questions were answered as the programme went along. It was extremely informative and well-structured throughout, all in all a fantastic opportunity that I am proud to have been a part of.
  – Medicine Calling Attendee 2020

- I found it interesting as there was a lot I didn't know before and it has definitely helped me consider what I'd like to do when I'm older.
  – Medicine Calling Attendee 2021

- The best thing was that we didn't talk to just one person about our ideas, but we talked to lots of different people (for example, students, doctors, nurses). This was a good thing as they all talked about their own point of view and helped me decide which career I might want to go onto in the future.
  – Medicine Calling Attendee 2022

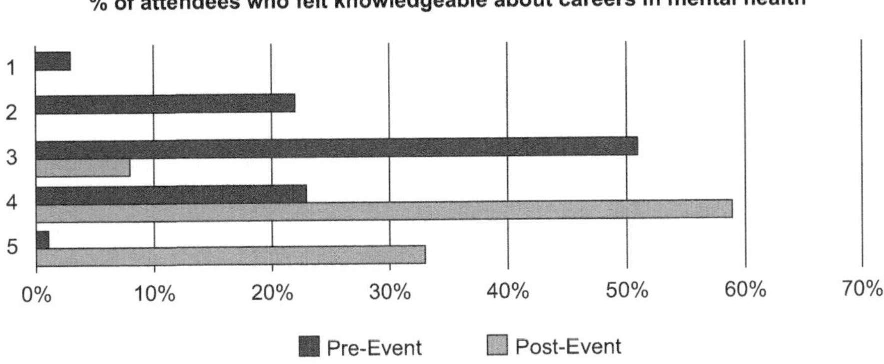

Figure 5.3 Graph to illustrate changes in knowledge of the variety of careers in mental health pre- and post-intervention

Conclusions

Since 2016, Medicine Calling has worked with more than 3,000 students, including a high proportion of students who are statistically the least likely to progress onto higher education. Our evaluations repeatedly demonstrate how students are more knowledgeable about careers in the mental health sector after attending a Medicine Calling event, and most importantly, students state that they are more likely to pursue a career in the mental health sector after attending an event. This demonstrates the value and importance of exposing young people to mental health careers with a view to attracting them to the sector and meeting the targets set out in future NHS workforce planning (NHS, 2023).

Throughout the project, Medicine Calling has overcome many challenges. For example, successfully targeting large number of students from widening participation backgrounds has, at times, been difficult especially during the Covid-19 pandemic. To combat this, Medicine Calling has worked closely with the central outreach team at the University of Leicester, who already have good relationships with local and regional schools and colleges. This has helped Medicine Calling to advertise its events to the most appropriate schools and colleges, ensuring they attract a diverse group of students and are well attended.

Additionally, we have continued to evolve the project over the years reacting to research and publications. This takes time and is not always easy when the majority of those who support Medicine Calling do this on a volunteer basis. For example, from 2018, the Medicine Calling team began to explore other influences on students' future career aspirations. For example, the influence that teachers, advisers, parents, and carers have on young people's career aspirations (House of Commons, 2023; Montacute and Cullinane, 2021; Mulcahy and Barrs, 2018). As a result, Medicine Calling developed talks and webinars, alongside our student events, for teachers and advisers to ensure they also have the knowledge to advise students about a range of mental health careers. In addition, Medicine Calling now engages with parents and carers. Medicine Calling invites parents and carers to accompany their son, daughter, or dependent to events to give them the opportunity to find out more about mental health careers, as well as take part in a dedicated parent and carer workshop to help them feel confident in supporting students with their future career aspirations.

Finally, it has not been possible to track all of the students who have attended Medicine Calling events to see if they eventually go onto a career in the sector. That said, the Medicine Calling team have met students currently studying at the University of Leicester, who have said they are studying medicine or mental health nursing as a result of being inspired at a Medicine Calling event which is extremely positive.

Implications

Although Medicine Calling is focused on careers in mental health, it could be used as a model for other specialties within medicine, as well as wider healthcare careers, to ensure more young people are attracted to careers in the sector. For example, the Medicine Calling team worked with staff at the University of Leicester to apply several of the same principles of Medicine Calling to a career in general practice, another area of focus in the NHS Long Term Workforce Plan (NHS, 2023). The University hosted two events for students in Years 9 and 10 called 'Careers in General Practice', which gave students the opportunity to take part in a range of interactive workshops, as well as meet a wide variety of healthcare professionals working in general practice. Similar findings, such as increased knowledge of the role of a general practitioner, and more students aspiring to a career in general practice, were found after the events.

Therefore, we argue that career-focused outreach and education around healthcare careers with young people should be an essential part of future NHS workforce planning. However, it is essential that similar projects focus on the schools and colleges they engage with to ensure they are supporting students from a range of different backgrounds, and students who are the least likely to have access to quality careers advice and guidance. This in turn could ensure the NHS is able to meet the targets set out in the recent NHS workforce plan in all areas (NHS, 2017), as well as helping to ensure the future NHS workforce is diverse and represents the society it serves.

References

Balon, R., Franchini, G., Freeman, P., Hassenfeld, I., Keshavan, M., and Yoder, E. (1999). Medical students' attitudes and views of psychiatry. *Academic Psychiatry*, 23(1), 30–36.
British Medical Association. (2020). Measuring progress. *Commitments to Support and Expand the Mental Health Workforce in England* [Internet]. www.bma.org.uk/media/2405/

bma-measuring-progress-of-commitments-for-mental-health-workforce-jan-2020.pdf (accessed July 2023)

Deb, T., and Lomax, A. (2014). Why don't more doctors choose a career in psychiatry? *British Medical Journal*, 348, f7714.

Dixon, R. P., Roberts, L. M., Lawrie, S., Jones, L. A., and Humphreys, M. S. (2008). Medical students' attitudes to psychiatric illness in primary care. *Medical Education*, 42(11), 1080–1087.

Henfrey, H. (2015). Psychiatry–Recruitment crisis or opportunity for change? *The British Journal of Psychiatry*, 207(1), 1–2.

House of Commons Education Committee. (2023). *Careers Education, Information, Advice and Guidance: Fourth Report of Session 2022–23* [Internet]. https://committees.parliament.uk/publications/40610/documents/198034/default/ (accessed July 2023)

Laugharne, R., Appiah-Poku, J., Laugharne, J., and Shankar, R. (2009). Attitudes toward psychiatry among final-year medical students in Kumasi Ghana. *Academic Psychiatry*, 33(1), 71–75.

Lyons, Z. (2013). Attitudes of medical students toward psychiatry and psychiatry as a career: A systematic review. *Academic Psychiatry*, 37(3), 150–157.

Montacute, R., and Cullinane, C. (2018). Sutton trust. *The Influence of Schools and Place on Admissions to Top Universities* [Internet]. www.suttontrust.com/wp-content/uploads/2019/12/AccesstoAdvantage-2018.pdf (accessed July 2021)

Morgan, L. J., Finn, G. M., and Tiffin, P. A. (2021). Are efforts to recruit to psychiatry closing the stable door after the horse has bolted? Knowledge and attitudes towards a career in psychiatry amongst secondary (high) school students: A UK-based cross-sectional survey. *Journal of Mental Health*, 17, 1–8. doi: 10.1080/09638237.2021.1922638. Epub ahead of print. PMID: 33999748.

Mukherjee, K., Maier, M., and Wessely, S. (2013). UK crisis in recruitment into psychiatric training. *Psychiatrist*, 37(6), 210–214.

Mulcahy, A., and Barrs, S. (2018). *Partners in Progression* [Internet]. www.cfey.org/wp-content/uploads/2018/07/Partners-in-Progression.-Engaging-parents-in-university-access.pdf (accessed February 2021)

NHS. (2017). *Stepping Forward to 20/21: The Mental Health Workforce Plan for England* [Internet]. www.hee.nhs.uk/sites/default/files/documents/Stepping%20forward%20to%20202021%20-%20The%20mental%20health%20workforce%20plan%20for%20england.pdf (accessed August 2020)

NHS. (2023). *NHS Long Term Workforce Plan* [Internet]. www.england.nhs.uk/wp-content/uploads/2023/06/nhs-long-term-workforce-plan-v1.1.pdf (accessed July 2023)

Palmer, W., Dodsworth, E., and Rolewicz, L. (2023). In train? Nuffield trust. *Progress on Mental Health Nurse Education* [Internet]. www.nhsconfed.org/system/files/2023-05/Mental-Health-nursing-update-in-train.pdf (accessed July 2023)

Royal College of Psychiatrists. (2020). *Psychiatrists See Alarming Rise in Patients Needing Urgent and Emergency Care and Forecast a 'Tsunami' of Mental Illness* [Internet]. www.rcpsych.ac.uk/news-and-features/latest-news/detail/2020/05/15/psychiatrists-see-alarming-rise-in-patients-needing-urgent-and-emergency-care (accessed August 2020)

Shields, G., Ng, R., Ventriglio, A., Castaldelli-Maia, J., Torales, J., and Bhugra, D. (2017). WPA position statement on recruitment in psychiatry. *World Psychiatry*, 16(1), 113–114.

White, E. H., Montacute, R., and Tibbs, L. (2022). Sutton trust. *Paving the Way: Careers Guidance in Secondary Schools* [Internet]. www.suttontrust.com/wp-content/uploads/2022/03/Paving-the-Way-1.pdf (accessed July 2023)

Appendix 1

Example programme: Year 10 and Year 11 Medicine Calling careers evening 2023

Year 10 and Year 11
Medicine Calling Careers Evening 2023
Programme
University of Leicester

16:45	Arrival and Registration
17:10	**Welcome and Introduction to Medicine Calling** *Discover more about some of the fascinating and rewarding careers connected to mental illness.*
17:30	**Empathy in Healthcare** *Find out more about the importance of empathy in healthcare, with a focus on patients with mental illness.*
17:50	**Break**
18:20	**Student Workshop** *Work with a healthcare professional to understand how healthcare professionals treat mental illness by looking at some case studies of patients treated during the Covid-19 pandemic.*
19:00	**What Do I Need for a Career in Mental Health?** *Find out what qualifications and skills you need to work in the healthcare sector.*
19:30	**End of Event** *Final questions*

Chapter 6

Widening participation of Aboriginal and Torres Strait Islanders in medicine

An international perspective

Louise Alldridge, Teleah Lindenberg, Maxine Hughes, and Glen Barry

Introduction

This chapter describes work conducted at a medical school in Queensland Australia just over ten years ago. Aboriginal and Torres Strait Islanders were and continue to be (thankfully to a lesser extent) under-represented in the Medical Profession in Australia. As stated by the Aboriginal human rights and social justice campaigner, Thomas Edwin Calma, 'It is not credible to suggest that one of the wealthiest nations in the world cannot solve a health crisis affecting less than 3% of its citizens.' In 2008, the Australian Government accepted what is now commonly known as the 'Bradley Review' (2008) which highlighted and exposed the significant under-representation of Indigenous students in Higher Education (HE) and set out recommendations to increase participation. The overarching aim was to achieve a proportion of Indigenous students in Higher Education that is equivalent to the Indigenous population.

The first Aboriginal Doctor graduated from the University of Western Australia in 1983, 14 years later there were 14 Indigenous Doctors. When this project was conceived in 2008, there were only 50 Indigenous Doctors in Australia. The under-representation of Indigenous Medical Students is a major contributory factor to the stark inequalities in health experienced by Indigenous Australians. These include increased death rate, decreased life expectancy, and increased infant mortality when compared to non-Indigenous Australians. At the onset of this initiative, the life expectancy at birth of Indigenous males was 11.5 years less than that of non-Indigenous males. Similarly, the life expectancy of Indigenous females was ten years less than non-Indigenous females (Australian Institute of Health, 2011). Shockingly, the infant mortality rates in 2006 were two times higher than for babies born to non-Indigenous women (Australian Bureau of

We would like to acknowledge Uncle Graham Dillon, Kombumerri Elder, Traditional Custodian and landowner of the Gold Coast for his leadership, wisdom, inspiration, and support. Without him none of this work would be possible.

DOI: 10.4324/9781003399858-6

Statistics, 2006). This is undoubtedly related to the low numbers of Indigenous Doctors as well as a deep-seated mistrust in the predominantly 'white' healthcare system as a consequence of the historical treatment by British Invaders in the past. The target to close the life expectancy gap by 2031 is not on track according to the recent publication by the Australian Government (National Indigenous Australian Agency Report, 2023). Priority actions still include supporting culturally safe and responsive Aboriginal community-controlled healthcare and increasing first nation healthcare workers.

The University and the Medical school had and continue to have a responsibility to challenge the consequences of the past and work towards an equitable future where access to education and to healthcare is achievable for all. At this time (2008), there were no alternative entry pathways or any targeted outreach or marketing for Aboriginal and Torres Strait Islanders to access Medicine at this University. The Medical School reserved five places each year for Aboriginal and/or Torres Strait Islanders, however, potential applicants were not overtly encouraged by their teachers, schools, and outreach or targeted by Medical School marketing strategies. All applicants for Medicine were expected to have high attainment in School, attain a high Grade Point Average (GPA) at university, and pass the Graduate Medical School Admission Test (GAMSAT) and selection interview. None of these admission tools were overtly culturally appropriate. The places did not generally get filled and were backfilled with traditional applicants.

Common barriers and solutions for inclusion of under-represented groups in medicine

Working as an educator in medical schools in England and Australia, it was clear that common barriers to accessing Medical Careers exist and persist for the under-represented groups despite significant differences in identity, culture, and backgrounds. Indigenous students and those from working-class backgrounds in the UK both lack basic educational opportunities, and face significant financial barriers as well as social and cultural barriers. Consequently, there is a paucity of role models, and they also develop similar negative attitudes towards their chances of success and belonging in Higher Education and Medicine. However, for students from Indigenous backgrounds, there are additional complexities, such as cultural fit, historical mistrust of 'white' Medicine, overt and shocking racism, and segregation. At the onset of this project, 1.1% of medical students in Australia were Indigenous (Ellender et al., 2008) whereas at this medical school the proportion was significantly less with only one student in all the four years, equating to less than 1%. At the time, the Indigenous population of Queensland was 3.6% of the state population. The reasons for this under-representation were and remain multiple and deep-seated in history. Selection and admission to medical schools were culturally biased and exclusive at this time. Negativity, open prejudiced towards

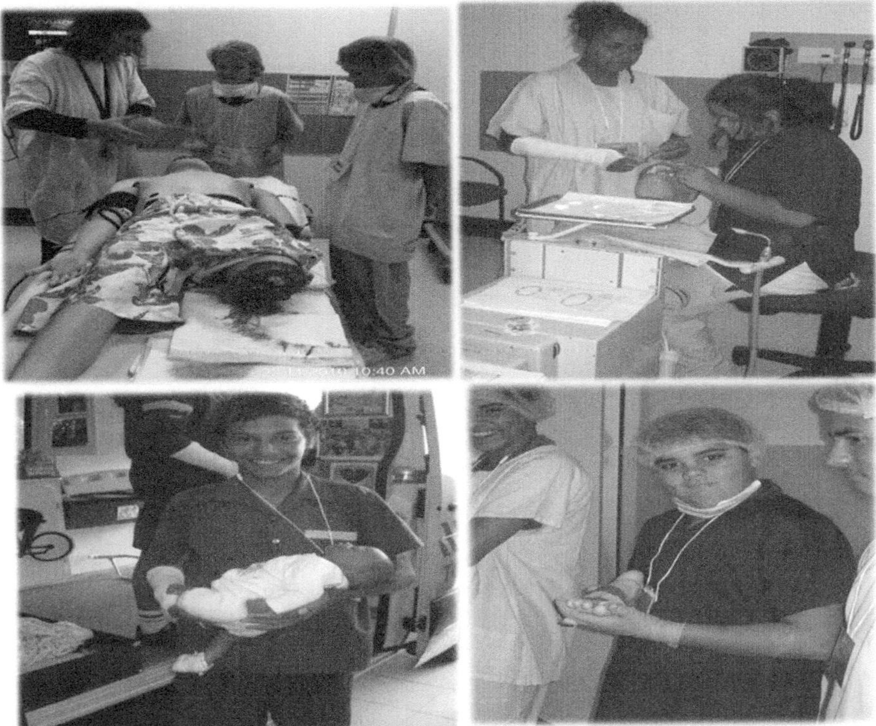

Figure 6.1 Barriers to and solutions for inclusion of under-represented groups in medicine

Indigenous applicants was also prevalent, and merit was seen to be predominantly racialised as 'white'. On top of this, and undoubtedly a consequence of the under-representation, Indigenous folk did not and to some extent still do not feel safe in a 'white, colonial' healthcare system, in fact the word hospital was used as a code word for the 'place you go to die'. The reasons for these feelings include colonisation (invasion), intergenerational trauma, and racism particularly in the healthcare system leading to second-class treatment.

It was clear that creating a pathway/s for local Indigenous students to access medical degrees was important not only for social mobility and inclusivity at the medical school but for equal health access, improved health outcomes of many Aboriginal and Torres Strait Islander people, and to fulfil a responsibility to challenge the consequence of the past.

The first step in this process was to connect with the community, inside and outside the University. We needed to identify and implement a strategy to support the aspirations of local Indigenous school pupils and encourage their teachers and families and community to see that a career in Medicine is achievable.

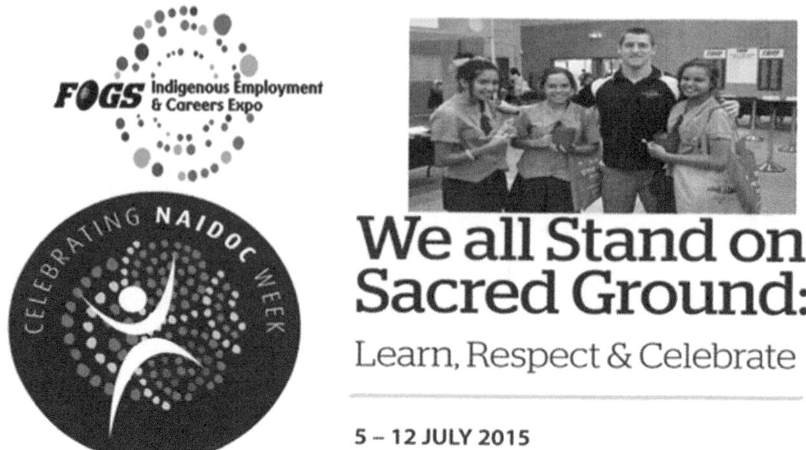

Figure 6.2 The first steps to widen participation of Indigenous communities

Griffith University has an Aboriginal Education Centre (GUMURRI). The centre is connected to schools and assists First Nation students to apply to the university and supports them up to graduation. Griffith University also has a resident Senior Elder who represents the Kombumerri people, the traditional owners of the land on which the University was built. The authors contacted the Senior Elder and explained the project and its aims. We were particularly grateful for his local knowledge which enabled us to access key schools and community group leaders and initiate a targeted outreach project to nurture the aspirations of local young Indigenous people and their families. The author was also encouraged to join local Indigenous 'yarning circles' where knowledge was shared, and respect was built. Such links to families and the community were key to the success of this project. The Senior Elder embraced the idea and helped the medical school by recommending and recruiting an Indigenous outreach officer to begin the outreach work in local schools with a high proportion of Indigenous pupils. The Senior Elder was also able to set up introductions to the only Aboriginal medical student in the school. This relationship with the Elder was pivotal to the success of all aspects of the project. The outreach officer was locally raised and embedded in the Indigenous community, full of energy and determined to change the face of Medicine in Queensland and is a co-author of this chapter.

Unfortunately, we were not successful in securing funding from the medical school budget at this time, however, we approached Education Queensland, the Local Education Authority, who welcomed the project and agreed to fund the outreach events and resources. Through this connection, we were also able to target and develop relationships with secondary schools with high proportion of Indigenous pupils and implement strategies to encourage and support their aspirations. During 'yarning circles', we were able to share our hopes and reassure the community that Medicine and Dentistry can be regarded as realistic and achievable career options. We also visited Head Teachers in schools to explain why the Medical School was keen to engage with Indigenous school children and build their aspirations to become Doctors. The project was named **Aspire, Realise, Achieve** with key objective to increase the uptake of Indigenous students at the School of Medicine and Dentistry using contacts in local schools and the local Indigenous community, identify 'role models', and build aspirations that will lead to good educational outcomes and a place at University.

During the first two years, we visited 32 schools and interacted with 300 Indigenous school children, 80 key workers including School Teachers, Principals, Guidance Officers, and Indigenous Community Associations such as Beenleigh Housing, Deadly Solutions, GPGC Kalwun (an Aboriginal community-controlled health and well-being community centre), Former Origin Greats (Indigenous Rugby League Players), and Black and Deadly youth group. School children were also invited to the medical school, where the only current Indigenous medical student at the time spoke openly about her 'story'. Following the key events, the outreach officer, who was closely connected to the local Indigenous people, was able to maintain continued contact with the pupils, their families, and schools.

Aboriginal and Torres Strait Islander Entry to Griffith University School of Medicine

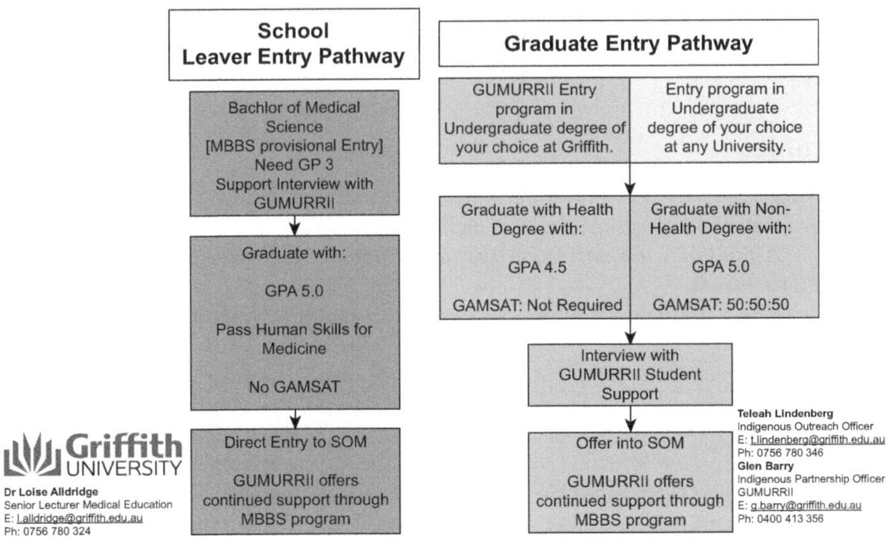

Figure 6.3 Outcomes of interventions

To improve the health and well-being of Indigenous Australia, we needed to grow the Indigenous Health Workforce. It was important to ensure we had at least one role model to inspire local Indigenous students. At the time, we only had one Aboriginal Medical Student. To mitigate this and increase our impact, we contacted the Dental School, where Aboriginal students were also under-represented. At the time, there was also only one Indigenous dental student, however, together they were successful in building aspirations for Aboriginal pupils to consider a career in Medicine or Dentistry.

Outreach work actively engaged pupils in activities and 'in-reach' visits to the medical school included talks from the two current Aboriginal students studying Medicine and Dentistry. This was followed by groups rotating through a variety of engaging clinical activity 'stations' including plaster casting 'broken' limbs, emergency care following a shark attack and Dental simulations.

Expansion and diversification of the outreach closely followed these 'in-reach' events. The outreach team took the message to other community activities, including NAIDOC week celebrations in our local community. These celebrations are held across the country to celebrate the history, culture, and achievements of Aboriginal and Torres Strait Islander people and are attended by Australians from all walks of life. This week is a great opportunity to participate in a range of activities and to support our local Aboriginal and Torres Strait Islander community. The outreach team attended many of these events to encourage attendees to consider Medicine and Dentistry as a realistic career. We also had a presence at the annual Rugby League FOGS (Former Origin Greats) events and recruitment stalls at the Rugby League State of Origin Game, as part of the Indigenous Employment and Careers Expo held in Brisbane and a 'Launch into Life' festival for School children in Logan, an area of Brisbane with high numbers of First Nation people.

Outcomes

> *The students received so much information that will guide them in making decisions for their immediate schooling as well as their future.*
> *A fun and informative day that left a lasting memory with our students, opening their minds.*
> Indigenous Support Coordinators commenting on the Activities Day

> *I never thought about being a doctor. I never thought I was smart enough. Now I do.*
> Year 10 pupil, Beenleigh State High School

The outcomes of this project were extensive and influenced life chances for many local Indigenous children alongside new aspects of teaching and learning in the Medical School curriculum.

Fairer access to a medical degree

These outreach events helped to build aspirations, raise awareness of the paucity of Aboriginal Doctors and aided pupils and teachers to realise the potential and realistic possibilities. However, navigating the complex and 'white' admissions and selection for Medicine remained a barrier for Aboriginal and Torres Strait Islander students. Working with the GUMURRII, the Medical Selections Officer and Lead for Selections and Equity (all authors) were able to devise alternative routes into Medicine and publicise the application process, eligibility, and criteria for Australian Aboriginal and Torres Strait Islander people.

At Griffith University, Medicine is a graduate entry degree, which provided a further barrier for Aboriginal Students as all candidates from all backgrounds were still required to have an undergraduate degree. The selection criteria at the time were comprised of three essential components: undergraduate degree, an Entrance Exam, and Interview. Applicants were required to achieve an overall Grade Point Average (GPA) of 5.0, which is equivalent to 65% to 74% in a bachelor's degree or other 'key degree'. They were also expected to perform well on a graduate admissions test, Graduate Medical School Admissions Test (GAMSAT), or the Medical College Admissions Test. Medical selections interviews were also a key selection tool (formerly Panel interview). Multi-mini-interviews were introduced by two of the authors in their capacity as Lead for Selection and Equity and Admissions Officer to mitigate for concerns regarding cultural incompatibility. These concerns persisted and culturally sensitive GUMURRII interviews were introduced for all Indigenous students accessing through this route. Furthermore, we introduced a multi mini-interview station assessing awareness and understanding of Aboriginal history into the direct entry interviews.

Further changes were made to make the selection more equitable for Indigenous student applicants and three pathways were devised. These included a pathway for school leavers, whereby students were able to apply to Griffith University with an OP3. These students were assessed through an interview conducted by Indigenous GUMURRII staff. They then studied for a degree at Griffith and upon gaining a GPA of 5.0 they were asked to take and pass an entrance exam known as 'Human Skills for Medicine'. The GAMSAT was removed due to cost of sitting the exam and at the time the exam was not culturally compatible.

GUMURRII offered continued support for all Aboriginal students studying Medicine.

For graduate Indigenous students, two linked pathways were available. If students had successfully completed a Bachelor of Medical Science degree at Griffith University through the Indigenous GUMURRII entry programme, they could enter Medicine with a GPA of 4.5 and again GAMSAT was not required. Students who had successfully completed a degree at any other university or a 'non' Health related degree were required to attain a GPA of 5.0 and to sit the GAMSAT exam and attain 50% or more in all three sections and perform well in the GUMURRII interview.

Table 6.1 shows the increase in number of students from Aboriginal and Torres Strait Island or Torres Strait Island origin enrolling in Medicine and Dentistry. The outreach work began around 2008 and the alternative entry routes were introduced in 2013. Although the numbers are not huge, there is a visible increase from 2014/15 when some of the pupils who engaged early on would have completed their school and degrees and been able to enter via the alternative routes.

Diversification of medical education

The outcomes from the engagement and activity were wide-ranging and generally positive for all the 'protagonists' in the story. Medical students gained meaningful and educational interactions with Indigenous Australian Children, their families, and Elders. This not only increased student and staff cultural awareness but also students were able to develop age and cultural communication skills vital for equitable care for their patients in the future. Staff and students also gained respect for the values and knowledge of Australian Aboriginal and Torres Strait Islander first people.

A further and much-welcomed outcome was the inclusion of Indigenous Health in the Medical Curriculum. Our connections with the community initially facilitated interactive sessions, including talks about the 'stolen generation' and the impact of separation on health and well-being for generations. Indigenous health questions were incorporated into assessments including a station in 2nd and 4th year Objective Structure Clinical Examinations. The First People's unit has now influenced the curriculum across all healthcare programmes, including remote placements in areas heavily populated by First Nation People such as the Palm Islands.

Progression: the first people unit

Both Indigenous co-authors progressed to prestigious university roles and were pivotal in the establishment of the First Peoples Unit for First Nations Students studying for a health degree. This unit now supports application, progression, and success in all university programmes and furthermore facilitates the integration of Aboriginal Health and knowledge into the teaching and learning across all healthcare degree programmes at the university.

Outreach has also flourished through the First Peoples Unit. Local Aboriginal school children attend university camps, to attain the full university experience, with emphasis on healthcare and health and well-being. Importantly, the unit also hosted students from rural and remote Aboriginal communities who were all inspired and believed they would be able to complete a health degree. Crucially essential financial support alongside tutoring has helped many

Table 6.1 Increase in Aboriginal and Torres Strait Island students enrolling in Medicine and Dentistry

Griffith – School of Medicine and Dentistry

List of students enrolled per year who identified themselves as being of Aboriginal original, or Aboriginal and Torres Strait Island origin, or Torres Strait Island origin

Doctor of Medicine + B Medicine/B Surgery

Student identification	2023	2022	2021	2020	2019	2018	2017	2016	2015	Total 2014	2013	2012	2011	2010	2009	2008	2007	2006
Of Aboriginal origin	5	10	8	12	11	11	11	11	10	7	2	1	1	1	1	2	1	1
Of Aboriginal and Torres Strait Island origin	3	4	4	4	2									1	1	1	1	
Of Torres Strait Island origin				1	1	1	1							1	1	1	1	
Total	8	14	12	17	14	12	12	11	10	7	2	1	1	3	3	4	3	1

Increased enrolment

students overcome significant barriers. This unit now works with each Health School at the University, providing further alternative entry routes with guaranteed places for a number of First Nation Students.

Factors critical for success

In this final section, we consider key factors that were critical to the success of this programme at the time. These factors can be applied across all widening participation work nationally and internationally. Many of the factors were implemented in a strategy in a UK medical school to enhance access and participation for under-represented groups, including care leavers, working-class/state-educated pupils, and refugees.

Overarching factors critical for success include targeted, holistic, sustained outreach linked to alternative routes into Medicine. Box 6.1 outlines a selection of important elements for success in this project that can be applied and adapted to most widening participation strategies.

Box 6.1 Factors critical for success

Understanding historical and present-day issues and the nature of under-representation.

Indigenous Outreach Officer who was fully connected to the local Indigenous people.

Connections with **and input** from Schools, Teachers/Friends/Family/Community/Indigenous Support Unit.

Dedication from Universities, teachers, community workers and/or Indigenous Support workers, and Outreach Workers who are engaged, effective, and connected.

Funding for outreach.

Targeted outreach that is inspirational/educational, informative from an early age, appropriate, and flexible.

Role models that are realistic, honest, and credible.

Education of Senior Managers, direct entry medical students, and medical and clinical educators.

Sustained support/mentoring: through **Indigenous Support Unit, Alternative entry,** Selection and Admissions pathway

Cultural and inclusive **pedagogy**.

Many of these factors are covered earlier, however, it is also crucial to understand the continued suffering that results from invasion and dispossession and the cruel removal of children from families (The Stolen Generation) which are unique to all Indigenous peoples (Korff, 2021) and have deep and long-lasting effects that are passed through generations.

In Gold Coast, its schools, and at Griffith University, there was a strong sense of Community for Indigenous people which is maintained today. Through the University's connections with the Senior Elder and GUMURRII, the Medical School was able to connect with key people and organisations. Appointing an Indigenous Outreach Officer was essential, not only for their enthusiasm and total investment in the cause but for the trust of the community, schools, and the pupils.

Many outreach projects fail to fully target those that are under-represented and often become conflated with marketing. A key to success at Griffith was to ensure every event was targeted and exclusive to local Indigenous pupils. Aboriginal students, Doctors, and Dentists who delivered outreach events and as such were also living, breathing 'role models' for the aspiring pupils.

To design any successful Widening Participation intervention, you need to understand the issues, know how to best inspire, and should employ relevant role models, preferably from the under-represented population. Outreach must be exclusively targeted to the under-represented population. It is also important to advocate for change by educating the senior managers and other staff and students. Most importantly medical educators should ensure an inclusive pedagogy, that is neither white nor classed, including assessment design and delivery. As Medical selections for admission is the first assessment for Medicine, inclusive changes were made to selections for this medical school, and these should also be passed on to the training stages of a clinical career.

Where are we now?

Significant progress has been made with the latest figures showing that last year (2022) 123 Indigenous students enrolled into Medicine. This figure equates to 3.53% of all domestic students enrolling into Medicine and has increased from 3.15% in 2021 and 2.7% in 2020 (source: medicaldeans.org.au). The numbers are now very close to the population of Aboriginal and Torres Strait Islander Indigenous population. Fifty-nine Aboriginal and Torres Strait Islander students graduated from Australian medical schools in 2022 (source: medicaldeans.org.au) and according to AIDA there were 757 Indigenous Doctors registered by the end of 2022.

These significant increases mean that there are now many more role models for Aboriginal and Torres Strait Islanders to send a very powerful message that helps them believe that it is possible to access a medical degree and become a Doctor in Australia. The knock-on effects of increasing the number of Indigenous Doctors include improved health and life expectancy. At the onset of the initiative, the average life expectancy for Aboriginal males was 56 and for white males it was Australians 77. This was unacceptable for two populations living in the same country with the same healthcare system. Currently, Aboriginal males have a life expectancy of 71 and white males have a life expectancy of 80. Other initiatives have been introduced to improve access to hospitals (Healthcare Spaces, 2022). Although there is still a discrepancy, the situation has improved for Aboriginal people and some of this must be due to the increased numbers of Aboriginal Doctors and increased trust and reduced racism in the Healthcare.

References

Australian Bureau of Statistics. (2006). *Experimental Estimates of Aboriginal and Torres Strait Islander Australians.* Canberra: Australian Bureau of Statistics. www.abs.gov.au/AUSSTATS/abs@.nsf/Lookup/3238.0.55.001Main+Features1Jun%202006

Australian Institute of Health and Welfare. (2011). *Life Expectancy and Mortality of Aboriginal and Torres Strait Islander People.* Cat. no. IHW 51. Canberra: AIHW. https://www.aihw.gov.au/getmedia/5e6b79b6-dbcd-45c6-a4d2-e5b5ce278ebc/12328.pdf?v=20230605180943&inline=true

Australian Bureau of Statistics. (2011). *Australian Social Trends.* www.abs.gov.au/AUSSTATS/abs@.nsf/Lookup/4102.0Main+Features10Mar+2011

Australian Government. (2023). Commonwealth closing the gap implementation plan. *National Indigenous Australian Agency.* www.niaa.gov.au/2023-commonwealth-closing-gap-implementation-plan

Bradley Review. (2008). *Australian Government, Department of Education, Employment and Workplace Relations.* http://hdl.voced.edu.au/10707/44384

Ellender, I., Drysdale, M., Chesters, J., Faulkner, S., Kelly, H., and Turnball, L. (2008). When dreams become nightmares: Why do Indigenous Australian medical students withdraw from the courses. *Australian Journal of Indigenous Education, 37.*

Healthcare Spaces. (2022). www.healthcare-spaces.com/2022/07/27/innovations-to-improve-access-to-hospital-care-for-first-nations-peoples/

Korff, J. (2021). Mortality and life expectancy of Indigenous Australians. *Australian Government.* Australian Institute of Health and Welfare.

National Indigenous Australian Agency Report. (2023). https://www.niaa.gov.au/resource-centre/niaa/2022-23-annual-report

Acknowledgements

Education Queensland, GUMURRII Centre, AIDA, IDA, Alamanda Private Hospital, Staff and students at Griffith University School of Medicine, Staff and students at Griffith University School of Oral Health, Equity Service Griffith University

I would particularly like to acknowledge the traditional owners of the lands upon which the five Griffith University campuses are located and pay respect to the spirit of the land and her people, the Yagarabul, Yuggera, Jagera, Turrbal, Yugambeh, and Kombumerri peoples.

Chapter 7

Different approaches to widening access programmes

Enam Haque, Jacqueline Higham, Sophie Hoyle, Alex Jackson (RIP), and Ben Ryan

This chapter is dedicated to the memory of a colleague and key contributor, Alex Jackson. Alex was the Access, Student Success, and Development Manager at the University of Manchester. He was an ally for our medical school widening participation (WP) team, providing his expertise and support to our work. An important project he supported us was the development of a masterclass for the Manchester Access Programme (MAP). This had been delivered during the pandemic as an online masterclass, but with Alex's assistance, it became an in-person MAP Masterclass Conference in June 2023. Alex sadly passed away suddenly in October 2023. He was only 40 years old. He leaves behind a wife and two small children. Our ongoing thoughts and prayers are for him and his family. He will be sorely missed.

Introduction

In this chapter, we look at the important contribution that widening access programmes make to improving admission to medical school for pupils from widening participation backgrounds. It does not cover other methods of gaining access to medical school, such as students transferring from other healthcare programmes or undertaking a graduate medical programme. It also does not cover the 'Gateway to Medicine' year, which enables students from WP backgrounds to complete a pre-medicine year at university, before embarking on the five-year course (Duenas et al., 2021). Pupils are selected onto these courses if they are from a WP background, and their curriculum varies between different medical schools. However, there is strong coverage of science subjects as well as modules to bring pupils up to speed on key qualities for medical school, such as study skills and professionalism.

Why are access programmes and similar initiatives so important? They break down the barriers to medical school for pupils from less privileged backgrounds. Those successfully completing these programmes are given a contextual offer to medical school. UCAS (2020) defined contextual offers as universities considering barriers that WP applicants may face and offering them reduced grade offers or special consideration for their courses. The Medical Schools Council (MSC) Selecting for Excellence Final Report (2014) highlighted the importance of contextual offers, to improve access to medical school. They advised

DOI: 10.4324/9781003399858-7

that this reduced the chances of pupils from WP backgrounds from missing out in the admissions process, while still ensuring that high-achieving pupils were enrolled onto the course.

The Covid-19 pandemic had a negative impact on this important work. In a questionnaire study by Bligh et al. (2021), they found that the pandemic markedly reduced pupils' opportunities to undertake work experience. However, virtual opportunities arose which mitigated a lot of these issues.

Three differing access programmes presented in this chapter as case studies highlight the different approaches to breaking down barriers for aspiring medical students. The first, Manchester Access Programme (MAP), is a nationally recognised programme, covering many different career paths. It is a source of pride for the University of Manchester, and the university has invested well on this. The medicine strand has been recognised as an excellent initiative by the GMC. Preston Widening Access programme (PWAP) differs, in that it is led by a team based in a Hospital Trust, with funding and support from a medical school. Volunteer medical students lead its activities, with the support of staff within the hospital trust. In contrast to these two programmes, Lancashire Access Medics (LAM) is a junior doctor led initiative in East Lancashire. It is affiliated to the University of Manchester, but is run as an independent, voluntary scheme. Despite all three initiatives being linked to the University of Manchester, their differing structure, organisation, and approach illustrate the diverse ways that aspiring medical students can successfully enter medical school.

Case studies

Manchester Access Programme (MAP) – Alex Jackson and Sophie Hoyle

The Manchester Access Programme (MAP) was set up in 2005 and has run since then as the University of Manchester's flagship widening access scheme. The aim is to support talented local students from backgrounds under-represented in higher education to progress to the University of Manchester or other research-intensive institutions. The scheme was set up as part of the drive to diversify the intake of universities and provide a pipeline of 'widening participation (WP)' background students.

Successful completion of the programme allows applicants access to a two A-level grade reduced offer onto undergraduate degrees, as well as eligibility for a bursary on enrolment at the University of Manchester, amongst other benefits.

MAP is celebrated internally within the institution, with support from senior leaders including annual representation at MAP graduation events by the Senior Leadership Team. The programme is also recognised nationally, with a formidable reputation across the higher education sector.

In its current format, MAP welcomes c.650 Year 12 students onto the programme each year. Within this, approximately 80 students will be on a Medicine-specific strand of MAP. The Medicine and Dentistry strands were created to support WP background applicants onto these highly selective courses. Only participants on the Medicine strand are eligible for the reduced grade offer for MB ChB Medicine at Manchester Medical School.

The exact requirements of completing MAP have changed over the years, particularly since the Covid-19 pandemic, but the core content remains the same. All students must complete four compulsory elements of the programme:

- Start Your Journey (programme launch)
- Academic Module: Research, Reference, Write
- Your Future Your Choice (attendance at a University of Manchester Open Day)
- Make Yourself a Success

As part of the Academic Module, students need to pass the Academic Assignment, which is a 1,500-word essay on a title of their choice. Each student is matched with an Academic Tutor who supports them one-to-one throughout the writing process. The University Life Conference was at one point a compulsory two-day event focusing on creating and delivering a group presentation using Enquiry-Based Learning, with a residential option. This has now been replaced by a summer 'Make Yourself a Success' event, to mirror the sector's increased focus on student success, although MAP has always been a programme that contributes to both access and student success.

Students are also able to attend a host of optional events delivered by the team. Amongst those are our Medicine-specific events: the yearly University Clinical Aptitude Test (UCAT) talk delivered by the UCAT team, and a Medicine and Dentistry Conference (previously the Medicine and Dentistry Simulation Day and Medicine Masterclasses), delivered in partnership with the Medicine WP Team. Students have the opportunity to come to the Stopford Building, where Medics are taught, and take part in a variety of workshops, including taking a patient history, ethics, how to save a life, and practice multiple mini-interviews. The day is facilitated not only by the Medicine WP Team and WP Fellows but also by Student Ambassadors currently studying Medicine, many of whom have done MAP themselves.

One student said,

[The] Medicine and Dentistry masterclasses were the best part [of MAP] as they gave the opportunity to talk to medicine students and medical workers. The sessions themselves were well organised and it was fun meeting and interacting with other students.

Since MAP began in 2005, 7433 students have completed the programme. Just under 3000 of those have been accepted on a course at the University of Manchester. Many other MAP graduates have been successful in obtaining a place at other research-intensive universities. In total, 341 MAP students have started a degree in Medicine at the University of Manchester. Of them, 199 have already graduated, 128 are currently studying, 1 student is on leave of absence, 1 student withdrew from the course, and 12 were removed from the programme (for several reasons). From all MAP alumni starting their degree in Medicine, only 2.6% of students have discontinued the programme (due to either withdrawing or being removed from the programme). Twenty-five students have been awarded a degree with Honours (including 5 with Distinction), and 174 students have been awarded an ordinary degree (including 4 with Distinction).

In 2023, MAP remains a mainstay of the University of Manchester's widening access offer. However, the programme has faced and overcome several different challenges over the years.

As with all face-to-face interventions, the national lockdowns in 2020 and subsequent elevated levels of restrictions in Greater Manchester presented logistical difficulties. All compulsory on-campus events were converted to online delivery, with c.650 college students joining the programme as planned six weeks after the first lockdown. Alongside this, the MAP team worked with the Medicine WP team to ensure that Medicine Masterclasses were adapted to Zoom-based delivery, with a new focus on discussion-based topics relevant to the cohort, such as taking a patient history, the principles of medical ethics, autonomy, and consent, how to save a life, and multiple mini-interview (MMI) skills.

By 2022 delivery, it became apparent that engagement on the programme, even with hybrid delivery, was suffering, with participants reporting 'Zoom fatigue'. The MAP team has therefore taken the learnings from online delivery to offer a blended approach, delivering events in person but with online catch-up opportunities for those who cannot attend. This provides greater flexibility for students who may need to travel from outer regions of Greater Manchester, such as Oldham and Wigan. This hybrid approach supports accessibility to the programme for students from low-income backgrounds, particularly with the cost of living crisis.

Looking to the future, the progression of MAP students through to undergraduate programmes will become more challenging. The changing population demographics will increase the number of applicants to university, with UCAS predicting that there will be one million applicants by the year 2030.

For applicants to Medicine, competition for places will continue to be fierce, with government restrictions on student numbers limiting intake whilst demand grows. For MAP students, the team is focusing additional attention on preparation activities such as an MMI session delivered by the heads of Medicine and Dentistry Admissions to try to mitigate the potential negative impact on their opportunities for progression.

In this sector context, it is likely that selective universities' ability to apply flexibility to entry requirements will be reduced in the coming years. The MAP team therefore maintains good working relationships with admissions colleagues, contributing to staff training around reduced grade offers and keeping lines of communication open. The team also offers a dedicated phone line for MAP participants to call on A-level results day, with the team offering additional advocacy on behalf of those with severe extenuating circumstances who have narrowly missed the conditions of their offer.

Many of our MAP students have now graduated and are working in Medicine. Dr Umair Gondal was a MAP student in 2010, Medicine undergraduate and MAP Student ambassador from 2011–2017, and now works as a GP in the north-west of England:

Participating in the Manchester Access Programme (MAP) in 2010 was a pivotal moment in my journey towards higher education. As a student who had moved from Germany to the UK in 2008, with limited knowledge of the UK education system and no family history of university attendance, I faced numerous challenges. MAP provided comprehensive support and guidance that transformed my academic trajectory.

Through MAP, I gained the necessary tools and self-belief to succeed and secured admission to medical school. Alongside my studies at medical school, I was a MAP ambassador and worked at events I previously benefitted from so much.

To this day I remember the interactive workshops on academic writing, study skills, personal statement writing and regular visits to the university. I enjoyed these a lot at the time and noticed when I started university it alleviated a lot of my concerns about fitting in as I was so familiar with staff and the campus.

The programme's impact extended beyond academics. I have lifelong friendships with fellow MAP participants, and even after 12 years, we maintain a close network that continues to uplift and inspire me.

Today, I work as a General Practitioner in the Northwest of England with an interest in medical education and leadership. I am deeply grateful for MAP's role in teaching me the values of mentoring and widening participation, which have shaped my personal and professional journey. Above all it broke that glass ceiling I often perceived I had when I first came to the UK.

Dr Sirat Lodhi was a MAP student in 2014 and commenced her studies in Medicine at the University of Manchester in 2015. She too was a MAP Student Ambassador, and is now working as an ENT Surgery Clinical Fellow at the Manchester Royal Infirmary:

I remember not knowing who to turn to for support with applying to medical school. No one in my family had been through this journey. As someone from a working-class background, I was also concerned about whether I would fit in at university.

The MAP removed my worries as I was immediately paired with a medical student mentor from the same background and had the opportunity to go through the application process with other students like me – students who had a lot of potential but lacked medical connections.

My mentor provided support with the application process. My university experience was significantly improved, all thanks to the MAP bursary. It allowed me to fund simple expenses such as medical equipment.

The support from MAP mentors and leads has continued to date and has supported my transition into beginning work as a doctor.

To date, I have completed an intercalated Master of Research degree, graduated from MMS, completed the academic foundation programme, and have commenced my current post at the Manchester Royal Infirmary as an ENT Surgery Clinical Fellow.

I attribute my successes to the MAP, as without the application guidance, mentorship, and the MAP bursary, I am certain I would not be in the position I am today.

PWAP – Jacqueline Higham and Dr Enam Haque

The Preston Widening Access Programme (PWAP) was established in 2014 and is aimed at supporting pupils from a widening participation background, who aspire to attain a place on the MB ChB programme at the University of Manchester. Pupils who meet WP contextual data requirements are often financially disadvantaged and struggle with the costs of going to university. PWAP provides opportunity for pupils meeting WP criteria within the Lancashire footprint the same benefits and opportunities as those students in the Greater Manchester area. Successful applicants from PWAP attend Lancashire Teaching Hospitals NHS Trust (LTH) in Years 3 to 5 for their placement years. This enables them to live at home and save on the financial burden of living away or travel expenses to the university.

The concept of an access programme is not new, with other Universities delivering programmes to aid candidates with their application onto a degree course. However, these programmes are delivered by the University and not at Hospitals. LTH is the first to deliver an access programme on a hospital site. PWAP was developed by LTH in collaboration with UoM (University of Manchester) and its structure was aligned with MAP. It comprises a range of activities and study that supports pupils to enhance their application to university. Pupils attend in-person biweekly workshops lasting three hours, held from January to July. All workshops take place at LTH and are delivered, facilitated, and organised by the LTH WP team, medical students, and doctors. Topics have been based on pre-existing WP activity at the University of Manchester and innovative ideas generated by medical students at LTH and current/former

PWAP attendees. The team delivers 13 workshops and topics include ethics in healthcare, interview skills, and confidentiality. Pupils are required to attend over 80% of workshops, gain 50 hours of volunteering experience, and author a 1,500-word essay to successfully complete PWAP. The essay provides them with insight into academic writing, including research and referencing skills.

Successful completion of the programme results in a guaranteed interview for a place on the MB ChB programme, with a slightly reduced academic entry requirement for successful applicants. The former PWAP attendee is then entitled to a bursary on enrolment. PWAP is part of UKWPMED, a collection of medical schools that recognise each other's access programmes.

In terms of impact, Health Education England (HEE) identified PWAP as an example of best practice and the GMC published its work. The programme is popular with local pupils, with 20–60 applications each year. In total, 249 pupils have attended PWAP since its inception, and we are proud to report an average completion rate of 75%. Most of these pupils were offered a place in medical school.

Many of our former PWAP pupils have now graduated and are practicing as doctors. Below is a testimony from one such PWAP graduate who feels that PWAP is 'life-changing':

Every Day I see the Benefits of the Programme.

Preston Widening Access Programme (PWAP) provides invaluable opportunities for those of underprivileged backgrounds to be given a chance of a lifetime. Children of disadvantaged backgrounds have many factors that limit their opportunity to become a medical professional, I know as I personally was a student on the PWAP programme and after having made friends throughout my medical student years, I really began to understand the value of the programme.

Pupils who are underprivileged can have a lack of support with their examinations and applications as well as a general understanding of the medical profession as a whole. They are more likely to do poorer in examinations and obtaining university admission in comparison to their peers who have parents with degrees, in the medical field or have a network of medical professionals. It meant many of my peers were able to get support from known medical professionals in their family with their examinations, interviews, and university applications. By being a student on PWAP I felt I was given an equal opportunity.

I am currently a second-year doctor, and every day I see the benefits of the programme. I also was a student on the programme and later became the chair of the programme. The programme trains students to become professional and obtain a deeper insight into the medical profession. It teaches students the role of a medical student, a doctor and also how to develop key interpersonal skills to work as a team to ultimately provide optimal patient care. It allows students to appreciate the demanding nature of the programme and prepare them in advance. It provides aid with communication skills and personal statements to ensure students are close to their peers (who have parents with degrees and higher education) in the standards of the application process for medicine alongside promoting professionalism. The programme is truly life changing.

The added benefits are that pupils from lower socioeconomic backgrounds later become surrounded by students of middle- and upper-class families, inevitably overtime resulting in a generational impact by allowing students to socially advance. In the long term, this can have remarkable societal and economic impact by increasing education, improving awareness, and minimising crimes which often correlate in those individuals of a deprived heritage.

Despite finding the application process really difficult, including A Level examination, I excelled exceptionally at medical school graduating with a honours degree. This made me feel that actually I was just as capable as my peers to become a doctor, which I previously doubted before admission.

Most of my peers were also from private and grammar schools which provide a surplus of resources and teaching to ensure maximal chances of entry onto medical courses for their students. The Statistics highlight this too.

Having PWAP as a college student, opened my mind and made me fall in love with the career even more. It allowed me to feel more prepared for medical school and life as a doctor.

We are proud of raising aspirations to local disadvantaged communities in Lancashire and look forward to many more years of developing the next generation of local doctors.

Lancashire Access Medics (LAM) – Dr Ben Ryan and Dr Enam Haque

The final case study highlights Lancashire Access Medics (LAM). This is a small programme founded in 2021 in East Lancashire, consisting of a team of junior doctor and medical student volunteers with support from the University of Manchester. They deliver an annual access programme to up to 20 sixth form pupils from WP backgrounds identified with widening WP flags in the Lancashire area.

The programme consists of regular online sessions, with an outcome-based curriculum. There are three phases to the programme, with each phase consisting of four sessions. These are outlined below:

Phase 1 provides an overview of the application process to medical school and life as a medical student and doctor. From this phase, pupils are expected to be able to create an effective and feasible plan to prepare for the different components of the medical school application process.

Phase 2 provides opportunities for pupils to develop key skills for medical students and doctors, through sessions on reflective practice, communication skills, and problem-based learning. Pupils should be able to write using Gibbs' reflective cycle, apply teamwork skills to group discussions, and employ professional communication skills when interviewing simulated patients.

Phase 3 focuses on the personal statement and medical school interviews. Pupils should be able to write an effective paragraph on a personal statement and answer common medical school interview questions with sound structure, reasoning, and communication skills. Topics are regularly revisited with increasing difficulty throughout, making it a spiral curriculum. (Masters and Gibbs, 2007)

Each individual session is designed to deliver clear learning outcomes which build towards the overall outcomes of each phase. Pupils' progress is assessed at the end of each session with a brief assignment, and students receive further support to achieve the learning outcomes if required. In this way, the programme uses constructive alignment (Loughlin et al., 2021) to ensure its outcomes, learning opportunities, and assessments are congruent.

The volunteers delivering the sessions are given clear guidance and training to plan their sessions, including how to apply Gagne's nine events of instruction (Gagné et al., 1992). This ensures that volunteers explore the pupils' prior knowledge on the topic and what they would like from the session, encouraging engagement and making the sessions student-centred. This also maintains standards throughout the project and makes it easier to support new volunteers.

Pupils' complete anonymous evaluation forms after each session exploring what they feel went well in the session and what could have been improved. For the 2022 programme, a focus group was conducted to explore what impact LAM had on pupils, and how it could have been improved. It was clear that the continuous support and student-centred approach had facilitated effective learning. It also highlighted that pupil wished for more support with their aptitude tests, and that the virtual learning environment was less engaging than being in-person.

One limitation in the evaluation process is that pupils have not historically been tracked to assess if there has been any impact on admission rates to medical school. The use of services such as HEAT (Higher Education Access Tracker) may facilitate this in the future.

In 2023, the LAM programme became accredited by the University of Manchester: pupils who sufficiently attended sessions and completed assignments, as well as a summer research project, were considered for lower UCAT and A-level grade requirements for admission to Manchester Medical School. Constructive alignment with clear and feasible learning outcomes is crucial for this volunteer-led access programme's success, who are limited by the time that they can contribute. Whilst the virtual-led approach means that volunteers can reach beyond the surrounding areas of medical schools, some pupils find it difficult to engage. This feasible and replicable approach may be successful in some respects, however, in-person sessions arranged locally, such as at hospital educational facilities, may be more engaging for students.

Future of access programmes

The case studies demonstrate that access programmes can be delivered both as funded and non-funded initiatives. However, in terms of sustainability, significant funding is required to ensure programmes do not die out when their creators leave. LAM has recognised this and has affiliated with PWAP to ensure there is administrative support for their work, as well as a coordinated access strategy in Lancashire.

Access programmes tend to serve the purpose of enabling local pupils from WP backgrounds to enter medical school, with a contextual offer. However, the question is whether this takes away opportunity and choice for them. UK-WPMed was created as a joint initiative between the National Medical Schools Widening Participation Forum (NMSWPF) and MSC Selection Alliance, to enable pupils with a contextual offer in one medical school to have the same contextual offer in another UK medical school (Haque et al., 2021). Developed by former deputy Head of Admissions at Keele Medical School, Dr Andy Spencer, this initiative has grown over the past few years to include seven medical schools. In 2023, it was officially adopted by the MSC Selection Alliance, as a key activity within its organisation. It is hoped that UKWPMed will expand, to enable pupils to have a wider choice of medical schools to attend.

References

Bligh, E. R., Courtney, E., Stirling, R., et al. (2021). Impact of the COVID-19 pandemic on UK medical school widening access schemes: Disruption, support and a virtual student led initiative. *BMC Medical Education*, 21, 344. doi: 10.1186/s12909-021-02770-0

Dueñas, A. N., Tiffin, P. A., and Finn, G. M. (2021). Understanding gateway to medicine programmes. *Clinical Teacher*, 18, 558–564. doi: 10.1111/tct.13368

Gagné, R. M., Briggs, L. J., and Wager, W. W. (1992, 4th ed.). *Principles of Instructional Design*. Fort Worth, TX: Harcourt Brace Jovanovich College Publishers.

Haque, E., Spencer, A., and Alldridge, L. (2021). Developing a UK widening participation forum. *The Clinical Teacher*, 18, 482–484. doi: 10.1111/tct.13357

Loughlin, C., Lygo-Baker, S., and Lindberg-Sand, Å. (2021). Reclaiming constructive alignment. *European Journal of Higher Education*, 11(2). doi: 10.1080/21568235.2020.1816197

Masters, K., and Gibbs, T. (2007). The spiral curriculum: Implications for online learning. *BMC Medical Education*, 7(1). doi: 10.1186/1472-6920-7-52

Medical Schools Council. (2014). *Selecting for Excellence Final Report*. selecting-for-excellence-final-report.pdf (medschools.ac.uk)

UCAS. (2020). *What is Contextual Admissions? What is Contextual Admissions? | Undergraduate | UCAS.*

Chapter 8

Transition of students from widening participation backgrounds to medical school

Identifying barriers and supporting success and progression

Nana Sartania and Clare Ray

Background

A successful transition is important for establishing a sense of belonging, subsequent student engagement, and academic accomplishments. Widening participation (WP) initiatives have increased the number of students from under-represented groups in medical cohorts nationally, but by definition they are still a minority, and this is likely to impact their sense of belonging as the majority of their fellow students will be more affluent and better connected. This chapter will discuss and critically evaluate the initiatives developed to support students from under-represented groups and the measures we think can be taken to nurture their sense of belonging at medical school. We believe that this is important for academic success and in establishing a fulfilling medical career after graduation.

While the approach to WP varies in the four nations of the UK, the majority of the medical schools use one or more of the following indicators to assess eligibility for contextual admissions and entitle a student to bespoke support measures where needed: attendance at a low participation school, being care experienced, refugee status, family estrangement, being in receipt of free school meals, or a resident in one of the 20% most deprived postcode areas in the country. Applying more than one WP flag for contextual admissions substantially improves the targeting of those who truly are multiply deprived. Using a blanket measure of postcode residence or the attendance of the low progression school alone will give an unfair advantage for some but would fail to admit applicants from target groups that should have benefitted from an adjusted offer. Students meeting the criteria and having participated in one of our WP programmes offered by Glasgow or Birmingham universities are guaranteed an interview and if successful at the interview, receive an offer typically 2–3 grades lower than the standard offer.

This chapter is not about widening access and implementing fair selection criteria to achieve the WP admissions goals. It rather builds on those and addresses the next stage: the successful integration of the WP students into medical school after admission. In an earlier paper (Sartania et al., 2021), we

DOI: 10.4324/9781003399858-8

identified the barriers that WP students themselves named in getting access to the medical school, and then being successful in it. Having identified the real and/or perceived social, economic, or cultural barriers, we will now discuss initiatives that can help overcome the challenges. Some of these are already practiced in one form or other by medical schools.

All students view transition from secondary to tertiary education as a challenge. In fact, they describe it as a 'culture shock' (McMillan, 2013), mainly due to anxiety about the challenges or disadvantages they may experience; they fear the new environment without old friends, feel alienated on campus, do not know what to expect and whom to turn to for help, and some feel homesick and lonely. Many WP students find it difficult to balance the demands of academic study with competing domestic and/or financial responsibilities at home and feel uncomfortable asking for help. The latter manifests in frequent trips home in the first term (if living away from the family home in university accommodation), which itself may perpetuate their loneliness and isolation at university, as they fail to quickly build their peer network when all the social groupings are being established. Commuter students may also experience similar isolation as they juggle their home and university lives. The 'culture shock' aspects are often exacerbated by higher academic standards required in the university (Pargetter, 2009; McMillan, 2013), busy first-term schedules (Larabi-Marie-Sainte et al., 2021), a lack of time to adapt to the new environment ('sink or swim' immediately), and the lack of support either from peers or staff to cultivate a sense of belonging (van Herpen et al., 2020; Sartania et al., 2021).

The challenge for a student is therefore to quickly adapt to the new environment, get to know their peers, and understand the university demands and expectations to assist their learning process. Failure to successfully manage such transition can lead to significant distress and poor grades (Picton et al., 2022), and increased drop-out rates (Yorke and Longden, 2004; Hassel and Ridout, 2017). An initial run of poor achievement reinforces the sense of not belonging in the medical school and undermines confidence further. It is often said that those with a higher level of emotional intelligence fare better in universities (Halimi et al., 2021), but then the emotional intelligence itself is linked to student's background, their upbringing, and the level of confidence the student will have (Schmalor et al., 2021).

It is reported by Briggs et al. (2012) that those who are the first generation in their family to go to university, and students from minority ethnic backgrounds, find the transition to university most difficult. While there are many reasons for this, one of the factors is often not knowing/understanding what the university expects of them, and not having the network to ask for helpful guidance. Staff may be genuinely approachable but may not realise the distance in status felt by a just-admitted WP student hesitant to ask 'stupid' questions that they fear everyone else probably knows the answers to.

Students are immediately expected to study effectively, but often insufficiently instructed in the skills to do so. Those from WP background are less prepared for the shift from school classrooms with the familiar, approachable teachers to the university's large class settings where the lecturers' expectation of students' work is different from what the pupils in secondary schools are accustomed to; comments like they 'don't know how to study', or 'how to find the resources' they can reliably learn from, have been quoted in the literature (Elliot and Bond, 2021; Sartania et al., 2021). The lack of 'privileged knowledge' was often mentioned in students' returns and this seems to permeate all the spheres from admissions to social interactions and networking. The combined sense of 'newness' and lack of clarity regarding what is expected of them (Yorke and Longden, 2004) is seen as 'frightening' and dampens their progress while raising anxiety.

Previous research reported that the students from higher socio-economic background are less likely to drop out of university and graduate with a 'good degree' (Crawford, 2014). The briefing paper on equality of access and outcomes in higher education in England (Bolton and Lewis, 2023) emphasises the need to reduce the attainment (or arguably the awarding) gap and provide sufficient advice and support both before and during the university, as well as help alleviate financial concerns that deter non-traditional applicants from applying and staying at universities. It talks about the need for the organisations to ensure that these students are valued for the different sets of social, cultural, and economic capital they accrue through their upbringing and different life journeys; and that they are provided with opportunities to grow in terms of their confidence to develop independent learning techniques and transition from 'not knowing how to study' to being fluent in a learning style that allows them to succeed at university. There are a few successful initiatives universities employ to help their students who fall in the widening access/widening participation category.

Pre-university interventions

While this chapter is about the experience in the transition phase in the first year of medical school, and how this can be tailored to increase the success and the sense of belonging for WP students, the transition is considerably eased when students enter with a better idea of what 'they are getting themselves in for'. Therefore, tailored pre-university interventions can have big impacts not just on recruitment and admission but on the transition too, and as such we will briefly address it below.

Since 2010, the University of Glasgow has run the Reach outreach programme. The initiative is sponsored by the Scottish Government and is designed to attract and raise aspirations in students attending schools with a progression rate below the national average. The pupils take part in the programme in the last two years of secondary education and attend 'in-school' or 'on-Campus' sessions that are designed to inspire, mentor, and guide those with the potential and ambition to study medicine, dentistry, veterinary medicine, or law.

While the aim of the programme is the same for each of the Scottish medical schools, each has autonomy on how their aim is achieved; as part of the effort, the Glasgow medical school trains and employs student ambassadors – themselves from similar backgrounds and admitted via contextual admissions – to deliver much of the outreach and help applicants with information on the admissions process, guide their personal statement writing, and train for interview during a week-long campus Summer School. They will also answer questions about the practicalities of studying at the medical school (e-mentoring). To date, as many as 1600 pupils from across the West of Scotland schools have completed the programme and more than 350 (>22%) of those have entered the medicine course in Glasgow, with others presumably entering other medical schools, in addition to dentistry, veterinary medicine, and other competitive courses. Another successful pre-entry programme in Glasgow is called 'Glasgow Essentials', acquainting offer holders with student life on Campus, assessment types, the university's virtual learning environment, and lessons on academic integrity. Once on the course, these students will have a welcome week where they can meet others from similar backgrounds to network and ask older students and staff engaged in the programme various questions about academic support or peer-enabled activities.

Similarly, at the University of Birmingham, 'Pathways to Birmingham' and specifically 'The Routes to the Profession: Medicine' programme works with Year 12 and Year 13 pupils from under-represented groups in the wider West Midlands, providing pre-application support such as mentoring, an opportunity to shadow current medical students at teaching sessions, work experience and simulation opportunities; the applicants are guaranteed access to an interview with bespoke preparation sessions leading to a contextual offer two to three grades below the standard requirement. Over the last three years, 15–20% of Year 1 students at Birmingham have entered via this route. Birmingham Medical School is part of the UKWPMED initiative, which originated from the National Medical Schools' Widening Participation Forum. This initiative includes seven Medical Schools: Birmingham, Brighton and Sussex, Hull-York, Keele, Leicester, Manchester, and Plymouth. These schools mutually recognize each other's Widening Participation (WP) programmes. Applicants who qualify under any of these programmes are guaranteed an interview at any participating school. If they pass the interview, they receive the same contextual offer as applicants from the WP programme of the school they applied to. This makes the 'WP consideration' portable and allows the students from WP background more choice in the schools they decide to apply to, while also being better prepared for their subsequent transition to their university of choice.

In university: approaches to teaching and learning

According to the Medical Schools Council's Selection Alliance, there are currently just over 9,000 medical students admitted annually across the 45 medical schools in the UK (MSC, 2024). Out of these, students from WP backgrounds admitted via contextual admissions now make up a sizeable group – between 5 and 40% (Garrud, 2024 personal communication), depending on a medical school's policy on widening access and the successes of their outreach activities. Currently, there are 19 medical schools across the UK that offer a bespoke, one-year-long Gateway course that prepares students for the first year of the medicine course. Such programmes provide tailored support and guidance to students throughout the year to ease their transition. Such bridging years do more than bringing the students up to speed knowledge-wise, but also bridge them towards the more academic (individual) style of teaching and learning with albeit less pressure than these students will experience in Year 1 of the medicine course. The bridging year allows students to feel like 'real' medical students right from the beginning when they are introduced to the concepts including professionalism, self-study, referencing style, and formative assessment.

Based on the limited research conducted, 42.9% of surveyed WP students in Glasgow found the course 'more challenging than non-WP students did' (Mirza and Rashid (2023). They felt under-equipped for transition and blamed the lack of academic confidence, financial hardship, and welfare issues as barriers for it. The suggestions offered to ameliorate the problem were to improve access to (higher levels of) financial support, to peer/welfare support resources, and to increase/improve training in academic skills such as note-taking during the transition phase.

Indeed, there are a number of steps that can be taken to help the incoming students from WP background transition from secondary school to the new experiences of university study. These all hinge on creating an environment where the students feel they can learn and where they feel they belong rather than suffer from 'imposter syndrome'. Thus, it is important to cultivate a sense of belonging and the feeling that all within the group have the same values (e.g., professionalism) and are united by the same identity (e.g., being a medical student of, for example, Glasgow University) or by having similar aspirations.

WP students need to feel they can achieve just as well as those from more affluent backgrounds. They need to have role models from the same background and need to be involved in communal activities where tasks are equally distributed to integrate better. In Glasgow, teaching methods are used that include collaborative learning (such as problem-based learning, case-based learning, or team-based learning). Students are asked to do work in groups (longitudinal portfolio coursework) that is assessed for community effort as well as individual contribution, making all students feel part of a group and strengthening bonds in a group where WP students feel included and involved. The need for mediators to be sensitive to group dynamics in such settings must be noted however, as students from WP backgrounds may feel intimidated by more confident peers. The group work may in fact play to the WP students' strength in some ways, as it is said that the relationship norms between the students from working-class backgrounds differ from those who are more privileged. Students from more affluent backgrounds are better prepared for independent, self-directed learning, while the cultural norm for those from widening participation backgrounds hinges more on interdependency and learning together (Manstead, 2018).

Glasgow runs various modules with the aim to nurture confidence and train students in academic skills. For example, one popular SSC module includes staff–student collaboration to write multiple-choice questions, and another to co-create educational resources. These modules have the potential for staff and students to contribute equally to course design and improvement and for staff to better understand students' experiences and perspectives – and vice versa. More importantly, participation in such SSCs equips students with skills they need for after university and develops higher levels of thinking in them. The experience teaches the students self-management and increases their engagement, while it helps to make the course more tailored to the needs, interests, and aims of the students. While these modules are open to all, students from WP background are particularly encouraged to take these up and the fact that many end up presenting their work at various educational conferences makes the modules popular. In addition to academic enrichment, this collaboration has a social function too and helps the students feel part of a community, including a direct (and much less formal) line of feedback to senior school staff – all empowering the students and facilitating confidence building.

Social dynamics between WP and non-WP cohorts

The implications of the difference in social and economic capital between WP students and the rest of the cohort go beyond the initial study skills and academic attainment. WP students often take up part-time jobs, leaving little leisure time to socialise. This can make social interactions and conversations awkward and even have the effect of making the WP student feel inferior. Moreover, this can become a restraint to speak up in non-social settings as well, for example, PBL or other group activities. As a set pattern is hard to overcome, the first weeks of transition really are critical in breaking these boundaries down, and more emphasis is needed on team-building and social interaction at that time.

Events that will allow informal networking will serve well at this stage. More attention needs to be given in the transition period to improving study skills, to managing the expectations, with emphasis on self-directed learning. This was one of the main barriers students from WP background identified as a major disadvantage compared to students coming from schools with high-participation rates in higher education (Sartania et al., 2021).

A study by Manstead (2018) explored whether social class does impact on not just behaviour but also thoughts and feelings. Fundamentally, members of the lower social class see themselves as more interdependent and have more empathy but as a result have greater difficulty to adapt to the essentially individualist learning experience at medical school, preferring group work instead. According to Manstead, these attributes largely stay with individuals, and this makes people from a working-class background less likely to apply to, be accepted by, or remain at workplaces where the middle-class style of independence is prevalent. There are no easy fixes to this but it is clear that 'imposter syndrome' is very real in the WP cohort and requires social rather than academic attention. Anxiety has effects on more than grades and can regrettably lead to an increasing number of students dropping out, affecting their professional development and mental health: the global prevalence rate of anxiety among medical students was reported as high as 33% (Dyrbye et al., 2006; Quek et al., 2019) and the picture is said to be no better for those students who fall under the WP category (Young et al., 2020).

One way to increase meaningful interaction between the WP and non-WP peer groups would be to introduce more project work for small groups, perhaps only three students, over a stretch of multiple weeks. It is essential that the task is authentic and requires collaboration and that the groups are randomly assigned rather than consist of already established social groups. Having a halfway report to class allows mediators to notice the group dynamics and participation. Such activities, when using peer assessment, do not need to be excessive with regard to staff time but could identify and perhaps even forestall dangerous isolation and anxiety in some students.

Widening Access to Medicine Student Societies (WAMS) networking events

Peer support can go and must go beyond mentoring by teaching and support staff. Student-led events, particularly important during Welcome Week (formerly Freshers' Week) can be an excellent way to support transition and start to engender a sense of belonging and enthusiasm. Traditionally, WAMS societies have been involved in outreach events to support access but increasingly they have highlighted the importance of supporting students from under-represented groups in navigating their time at university. Example of this are the networking events, run by both the Birmingham WAMS and the Glasgow WAMS, early in the first term, which give students from WP backgrounds the opportunity to come together in a friendly and social setting (preferably with food and drink provided) to meet one another, as well as students from later years and key members of staff they will be interacting with throughout the first year of study. During the events, Birmingham WAMS lead some fun networking activities and quizzes and also, a cross-year Q & A panel with representatives from all year groups so that new Year 1 students have the opportunity to ask questions they have about the entire duration of the course and hear different students' perspectives and experiences. The participants value the opportunity to make connections with one another, especially those who did not take part in University's access programme. In Glasgow various social events such as welcome lunches, Christmas lunches, and drop-in sessions with students from all years of the course provide opportunities for incoming students to meet 'older' students and integrate into the existing network.

Establishing a social network via a WP student society is an efficient way of cultivating a sense of belonging; students can engage in community work (for example, take part in outreach, help with Summer Schools, or help organise networking events for freshers), and develop a sense of shared responsibility for the welfare of others from a similar background; the additional benefit of informal interaction between staff and students, as well as between the WP students at all stages of their education cannot be underestimated as an outcome of the WAMS – all these fit well into the medical ethos that students are expected to develop over the same years.

Suggestions to combat 'imposter syndrome'

Academic services in supporting transition and belonging

Support for the development of belonging skills can be important to build students' confidence in their abilities, engage more fully in academic teaching activities (e.g., tutorials and group learning sessions), and increase sense of belonging by addressing some of the factors that contribute to imposter syndrome. Library support services, including the Academic Skills Centre at the University of Birmingham and the Student Learning Development at the University of Glasgow, provide support for any student wishing to develop their academic skills or who might require support with a particular element of their academic work (including note-taking, writing, mathematics, critical analysis, and organisational skills). In Birmingham, as part of the commitment to widening participation through the *Access and Participation Plan*, students from WP backgrounds are entitled to enhanced support from these services, including an increased number of one-to-one appointments with effective learning advisers. However, this still requires the students to actively seek such help, and it may be the less extrovert and less confident students that need it the most. As such, study skills teaching for everyone should be enhanced in the first weeks of transition, including approaches to different teaching sessions (interactive sessions, lectures, tutorials, and PBLs), small group work on finding specific information through library and online searches, structured teaching on referencing, different assessment styles, and types of feedback.

Enhanced Personal Academic Tutoring (PAT)

At Birmingham, students from WP backgrounds are also able to access enhanced personal academic tutoring (PAT; equivalent to the 'Advisors of Study' scheme in Glasgow) with up to three additional tutor meetings per year. This provision aims to address the disadvantage of a lower level of social and cultural capital that students from a widening participation background might have. Personal academic tutors are also able to refer students directly to support and enhancement services helping students to navigate the university systems more easily – crucial when many students are having to work part-time (and even full time) to support their studies and therefore are chronically short on study time. The widespread initiative by Med Socs to assign peer mentors to new students from WP backgrounds is a welcome addition to the safety net for the incoming students and alongside the existing central university support and welfare services help with transition. This system might be further enhanced by staff working with Med Socs to ensure that they have the training and information they need to ensure they also engender an inclusive environment.

Financial support to help with transition and sense of belonging

The feelings of 'not fitting in' for WP students are exacerbated by the acquisition of different or more accurately 'unmatched' social or cultural capital, but also by the lack of economic capital (Friedman and Laurison, 2019). These students may not have access to sufficient financial support beyond that provided by student finance, and often need to work part-time (or more) to support themselves and also to contribute to their family's finances – potentially leaving them too tired and too short of time to socialise, having to spend their available hours on academic work. This situation leads to the perpetuation of their social capital deficit and further isolation and feeling behind with their studies.

The hidden costs of studying for a medical degree (including, for example, transport, equipment, and clothing) combined with longer contact teaching hours and academic terms, and the length of the medical programmes, means that the financial disadvantage is likewise compounded. As well as the direct financial impact of limited resources, the time cost of worrying about money and, for instance, applying for additional funding or reclaiming travel costs, puts students at a disadvantage as they will have less time to dedicate to their academic work and less time to participate in extra- and co-curricular activities that would have enhanced their time at university and allowed them to develop the social and cultural capital to improve their career prospects. It would serve many benefits if these students could have paid employment by universities or be offered a start-up grant at the start of the transition phase – as is the case in Southampton or Aberdeen. Equally, an initiative by the University of Edinburgh to employ medical school undergraduate scholars to support WP students on the course and then feedback to medical school about the issues the students face on the course or on placements should be replicated by many.

Access to additional financial support can really be important in providing students with the financial security and peace of mind that is essential for them to focus on their studies and access extracurricular activities (Sartania, 2023). Many universities offer financial support to students who have completed their own widening participation programme with a scholarship or bursary paid annually (Birmingham, Southampton, St Georges, and Aberdeen). Universities often also offer a means-tested scholarship or bursary based on household income. This is an area of support that could be developed further.

Universities offer financial support for students in need – via university hardship and discretionary funds. However, many students have reported that the application process for this type of support can be very intrusive, requiring students to provide detailed breakdowns of their income and spending. This in itself can take a lot of time for students who are already time poor. On a more positive note, the number of scholarships and grants available that are supported by generous donations and bequests of alumni and other benefactors are now being targeted at students from WP background and other under-represented groups (e.g., scholarships for African/Afro-Caribbean origin). There is, however, no doubt that the cognitive burden of worrying about finances is another barrier that students from socio-economically disadvantaged backgrounds have to deal with, taking time that their more advantaged peers can dedicate to academic study or other activities which may ultimately improve their prospects. Ideally, every WP student in need of financial support should get a means-tested bursary from the government to negate the necessity for working long hours during term-time, so the students can concentrate on succeeding and progressing well on the course and graduating without delay.

The role of co-curricular and extracurricular activities in supporting transition and sense of belonging

WP students are often reluctant to take up co- and/or extracurricular activities as they see no immediate benefit of investing time and finances in them. However, these activities have a large role to play in engendering a sense of belonging and, equally importantly, in giving students the opportunity to engage with a range of experiences that will support their professional development and impact their career prospects. For example, although now not taken into consideration for Foundation placement, a student's engagement with research, any work experience placements or internships, intercalated degrees, or the opportunity to travel during electives, all promote personal and professional development that will impact a doctor's career progression.

Financial barriers put students from a WP background at an unfair disadvantage when it comes to accessing additional activities. Birmingham has gone some way towards addressing this by offering bursaries to intercalating students from WP backgrounds. The Birmingham WAMS society also runs an annual event, a Research Rodeo, which gives students from a WP background early information about the benefits of getting involved with these co-curricular activities and provides networking opportunities to support them to identify placements. In Glasgow, a student society called GUMRS (Glasgow University Medical Research Society) runs various training workshops and offers students opportunities to take part in research studies or audits. While students from WP background may well be aware of the benefit of such activities, they may not engage due to time constraints and financial reasons. A large proportion of students from WP background will choose not to intercalate for the same reason, meaning they miss out on academic enrichment opportunities.

Accessing extracurricular activities including clubs and societies can also be prohibitively expensive and such organisations often do not cater for students living away from campus or its immediate area. Students are aware of the importance of these activities for their physical and mental well-being including the opportunity to network, but often a significant proportion of the student population is excluded. This may lead to setting up a two-tier system and a cohort where sense of belonging is adversely impacted leading to potential attainment/awarding gaps and diminished student well-being and satisfaction. Ensuring that Student Unions and Guilds are aware of the challenges that different students face, and are supported to provide training in equality, diversity and inclusivity to society committees, this may start to address some of the issues.

Conclusion

In summary, all students find transition to university life difficult, but the challenges tend to be exacerbated in students from groups under-represented in higher education. Failure to recognise this can lead to poor academic outcomes and poor mental health. Medical schools should strive to recognise early signs of isolation and challenge them by providing initiatives designed to cultivate a culture of support and acceptance/inclusivity; the measures currently in place to support student transition include community building, feeling like a 'real' medical student (sense of belonging), supporting study skills, and providing pastoral support. While many of these are in practice and being refined by schools with a positive ethos of widening access and participation, there is more to be done, especially in ensuring financial security for these students.

References

Bolton, P., and Lewis, J. (2023, January 31). Equality of access and outcomes in higher education in England. *House of Commons Library*. https://commonslibrary.parliament.uk/research-briefings/cbp-9195/#:~:text=on%20this%20measure.-,Socio%2Deconomic%20status,second%20year%20in%20higher%20education (accessed 4 January 2024)

Briggs, A. R. J., Clark, J., and Hall, I. (2012). Building bridges: Understanding student transition to university. *Quality in Higher Education*, 18(1), 3–21. doi: 10.1080/13538322.2011.614468

Crawford, C. (2014). *Socio-economic differences in university outcomes in the UK: Drop-out, degree completion and degree class*. Institute for Fiscal Studies Working Paper. https://ifs.org.uk/publications/socio-economic-differences-university-outcomes-uk-drop-out-degree-completion-and (accessed 15 May 2024)

Dyrbye, L. N., Thomas, M. R., and Shanafelt, T. D. (2006). Systematic review of depression, anxiety and other indicators of physiological distress among US and Canadian medical students. *Academic Medicine*, 81, 354–373. doi: 10.1097/00001888-200604000-00009

Elliot, M., and Bond, D. (2021). www.futurelearn.com/courses/skills-to-succeed-at-university

Friedman, S., and Laurison, D. (2019). *The Class Ceiling: Why it Pays to be Privileged*. Policy Press. doi: 10.2307/j.ctv5zftbj

Halimi, F., AlShammari, I., and Navarro, C. (2021). Emotional intelligence and academic achievement in higher education. *Journal of Applied Research in Higher Education*, 13(2), 485–503. doi: 10.1108/JARHE-11-2019-0286

Hassel, S., and Ridout, N. (2018). An investigation of first-year students' and lecturers' expectations of University education. *Frontiers in Psychology*, 26(8), 2218. doi: 10.3389/fpsyg.2017.02218

Larabi-Marie-Sainte, S., Jan, R., Al-Matouq, A., and Alabduhadi, S. (2021). The impact of timetable on student's absences and performance. *PLoS One*, 16(6), e0253256. doi: 10.1371/journal.pone.0253256

Manstead, A. S. R. (2018). The psychology of social class: How socioeconomic status impacts thought, feelings, and behaviour. *British Journal of Social Psychology* 57(2), 267–291. doi: 10.1111/bjso.12251

McMillan, W. (2013). Transition to university: The role played by emotion. *European Journal of Dental Education*, 7(3), 169–176.

Medical Schools A-Z. in Medical schools | Medical Schools Council. medschools.ac.uk. (accessed 1 February 2024)

Mirza, S., and Rashid, A. (2023). Aiding transition of widening participation students post university admissions. *Poster Presented at the 5th Conference of the National Medical Schools Widening Participation Forum*, Birmingham.

Pargetter, R. (2009). Transition: From a school perspective. *Journal of Institutional Research*, 2000(9), 14–21.

Picton, A., Greenfield, S., and Parry, J. (2022). Why do students struggle in their first year of medical school? A qualitative study of student voices. *BMC Medical Education*, 22, 100. doi: 10.1186/s12909-022-03158-4

Quek, T. T., Tamm, W. W., Tran, B. X., Zhang, M., Zhang, Z., Ho, C. S., and Ho, R. C. (2019). The global prevalence of anxiety among medical students: A meta-analysis. *International Journal of Environmental Research and Public Health*, 16(15), 2735. doi: 10.3390/ijerph16152735. PMID: 31370266: PMCID: PMC6696211.

Sartania, N. (2023). Admissions to medical school is not the endpoint of widening participation. *oSoTL*, 2(3), 19–29. ISSN 2752–4116.

Sartania, N., Alldridge, L., and Ray, C. (2021). Barriers to access, transition and progression of widening participation students in UK medical schools: The students' perspective. *MedEdPublish*, 10, 132. doi: 10.15694/mep.2021.000132.1

Schmalor, A., Cheung, B. Y., and Heine, S. J. (2021). Exploring people's thoughts about the causes of ethnic stereotypes. *PLoS One*, 16(1), e0245517. doi: 10.1371/journal.pone.0245517

van Herpen, S. G. A., Meeuwisse, M., Hofman, W. H. A., and Severiens, S. E. (2020). A head start in higher education: The effect of a transition intervention on interaction, sense of belonging, and academic performance. *Studies in Higher Education*, 45(4), 862–877. doi: 10.1080/03075079.2019.1572088

Yorke, M., and Longden, B. (2004). *Retention and student success in higher education*. Society for Research into Higher Education & Open University Press.

Young, E., Thomson, R., Sharp, J., and Bosmans, D. (2020). Emotional transitions? Exploring the student experience of entering higher education in a widening participation HE-in-FE setting. *Journal of Further and Higher Education*, 44(10), 1349–1363. doi: 10.1080/0309877X.2019.1688264

National project to address under-representation of students from disadvantaged backgrounds

Paul Garrud, Clare Owen, and Ceri Nursaw

Background

In their 2012 report (Milburn, 2012), the Social Mobility and Child Poverty Commission said, *'medicine lags behind other professions both in the focus and in the priority, it accords to'* (widening participation – WP). *'It has a long way to go when it comes to making access fairer, diversifying its workforce and raising social mobility.'* This trenchant challenge, combined with evidence about variation in recruitment and selection of medical students, led to the establishment of the 'Selecting for Excellence' project, involving key stakeholders (UK government, professional regulator, workforce organisations, social mobility charities, higher education bodies, and medical schools).

Their final report (SMCPC, 2014) summarised the data about the considerable under-representation of young people from disadvantaged backgrounds amongst applicants and entrants to medical school, as well as trainees in medicine post-qualification. Figure 9.1 depicts several facets of socio-economic disadvantage indicating that the majority come from professional and managerial backgrounds and geographical areas with high progression to higher education (HE).

The SfE final report (MSC, 2014) made substantial recommendations for change directed at each of its stakeholders, including individual medical schools and Medical Schools Council (MSC), that represents all UK medical schools at the national level. In response, MSC set up a Selection Alliance to implement these changes, with representation from all UK medical schools and suitable governance and oversight processes.

Change management

MSC is a membership organisation and in the SfE project, followed current best practice in stakeholder engagement (Jeffery, 2009; Kezar, 2023). In particular, by facilitating the involvement of those potentially affected by or interested in widening access (WA) and participation (WP), recognising and communicating the needs and interests of all participants, and ensuring that

DOI: 10.4324/9781003399858-9

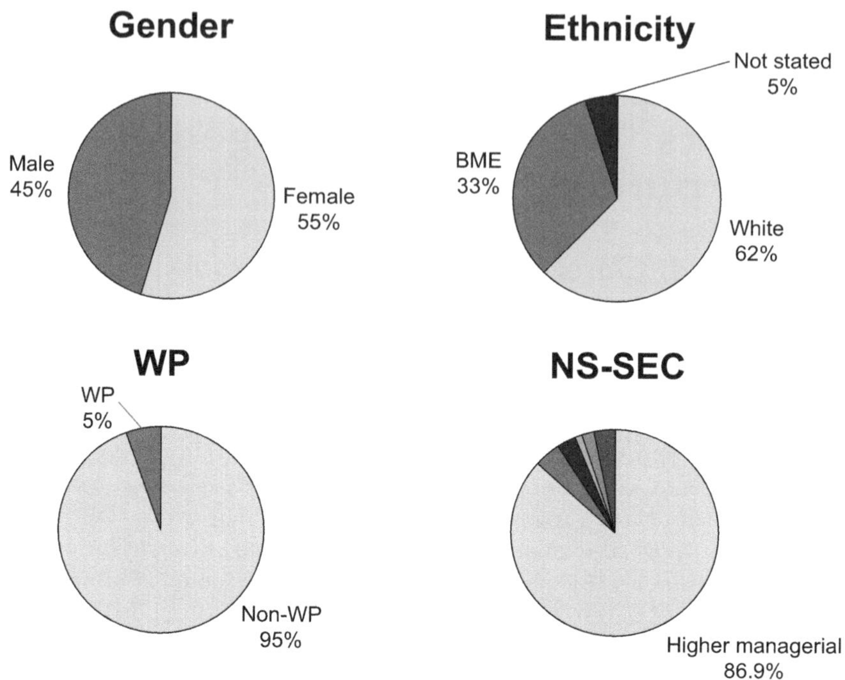

Figure 9.1 Medical Schools Annual GMC Return 2014 (BME: Black, Asian and Minority Ethnicity; WP: POLAR 1 quintile, non-WP quintiles 2–5; NS-SEC: National Statistics Socio-economic Classification)[1]

stakeholders had a say in decisions about recommendations to widen participation in medicine.

In the work reported below, this aspect of SfE was addressed, in part, with outreach activities involving student WP groups and secondary schools and colleges; however, it's clear that the broader population of potential WP students have had little input or engagement as stakeholders, though they have participated in a wide variety of outreach.

Another requirement of best practice is to facilitate alignment or, where need be, agreed consensus between stakeholders. In several respects, alignment has been good and maintained over ten years at governmental level, in healthcare workforce planning, and by medical schools, with the broad agreement of two principles:

- That awareness, preparation, application, and entry to medical school (and, thus, the medical profession) should be equitable across different degrees of disadvantage;[2]
- That a diverse healthcare workforce that fully represents the population it serves will provide a higher quality of care.

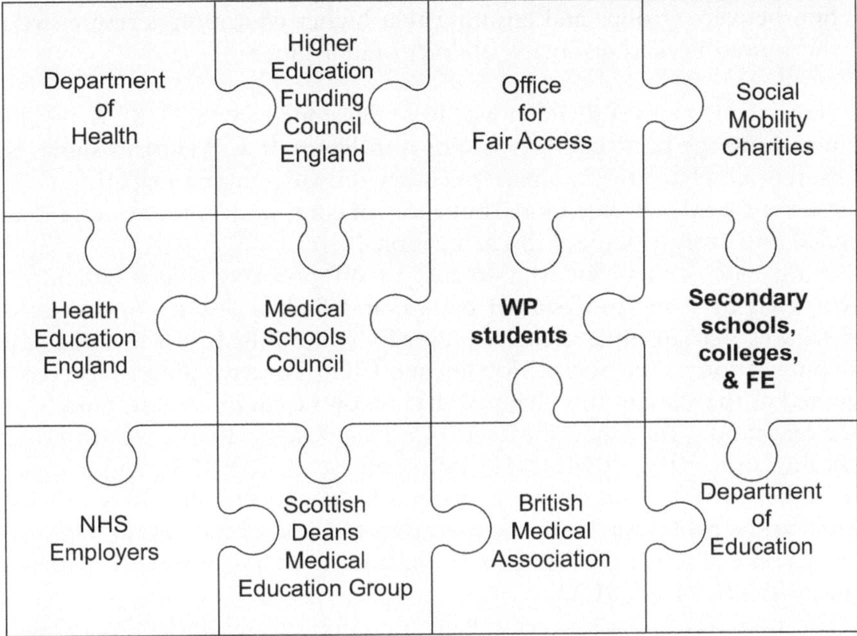

Figure 9.2 Stakeholder organisations represented (black) in Selecting for Excellence; unrepresented groups (red)

One factor, where compromise existed prior to SfE and still continues, is the strong need for additional fee income in medical schools, most often from international students, but also from private students (self-funded, not state-supported). Current estimates are that around 7.5% of medical school places are filled in this way (OfS, 2023).

The Alliance has continued with a philosophy of stakeholder engagement, using its membership (two representatives from each medical school, usually including the admissions dean/tutor), governance (an elected board), reporting (an annual report plus an annual Oversight Group made up of the original SfE stakeholders, or their replacement bodies), and support of student WP groups and the National Medical Schools WP Forum.

Integrated and coordinated action

The Dearing Report (HMSO, 1997) initiated the priority of widening participation in UK higher education; it stated:

increasing participation in higher education is a necessary and desirable objective of national policy over the next 20 years. This must be accompanied by the objective of reducing the disparities in participation in higher education between groups and ensuring that higher education is responsive to the aspirations and distinctive abilities of individuals.

Since then, many WP initiatives have developed in the UK. A timeline summarising the principal ones is shown in Figure 9.3. What this shows is a consistent emphasis over a quarter century on widening participation in HE across the four devolved nations, but a lack of continuity in the structures and funded initiatives to achieve this at a national level.

In the case of medicine, the urgency of WP probably lagged behind, unrecognised by many professional bodies, and finding less traction in medical schools than in other areas of university education. It was in 2012, with the publication of the Social Mobility and Child Poverty Commission report (quoted at the start of this chapter) that action began in earnest. Since then, medical schools, the General Medical Council (GMC, 2016), Health Education England (HEE, 2014), NHS Education Scotland (NES), and comparable bodies in Wales and Northern Ireland have worked collectively to widen access to the profession, with support from HE bodies such as the Office for Fair Access and Office for Students in England, and Universities Scotland (e.g. Universities Scotland, 2023).

This past decade has also seen the recognition of substantial threats to the NHS workforce (including doctors), with concerns about shortage specialties such as general practice (BMA, 2023), psychiatry, and acute medicine, as well as geographical shortages (e.g., inner cities, remote and rural areas, and coastal towns). This in turn has led to stronger involvement of specialty bodies – many Royal Colleges and specialty societies – in pre-university outreach as well as working with current medical students (examples are discussed further on).

Thus, one important national challenge has been to co-ordinate the work of multiple organisations (stakeholders) in this sector. That challenge has only been met in part for two main reasons: first, that no one organisation has an overarching responsibility for WP and there is no umbrella structure to link their WP efforts, and second, that each individual organisation has conflicting demands for its resources (if not, sometimes, perverse incentives, or absolute boundaries).

In addition to the national challenge, when one considers WP activity at regional and local levels, co-ordination has often been a lost cause. Similar projects in different areas may duplicate each other's work and remain unaware of existing resources or evidence about what works and what doesn't.

The response to this has been attempts to network people and organisations working in the sector (an example in medicine is the National Medical Schools WP Forum, or across HE Uni Connect[3] and NEON[4]), but this has had limited reach.

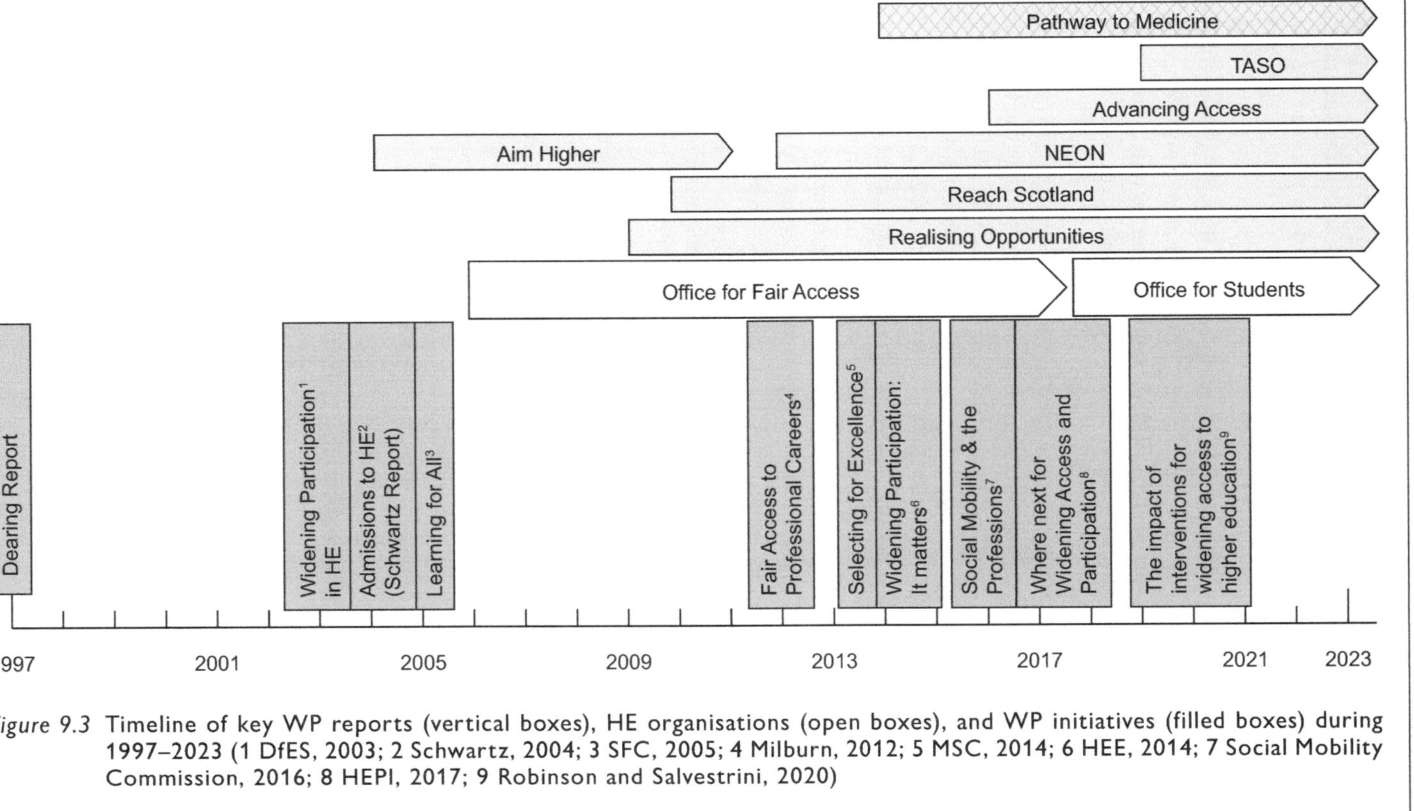

Figure 9.3 Timeline of key WP reports (vertical boxes), HE organisations (open boxes), and WP initiatives (filled boxes) during 1997–2023 (1 DfES, 2003; 2 Schwartz, 2004; 3 SFC, 2005; 4 Milburn, 2012; 5 MSC, 2014; 6 HEE, 2014; 7 Social Mobility Commission, 2016; 8 HEPI, 2017; 9 Robinson and Salvestrini, 2020)

There have been many national initiatives, several of which have proved not just successful, but also influential – facilitating dissemination and take-up beyond their initial constituency. One example is work supported by the Royal College of General Practitioners (Nicholls et al., 2012; RCGP, 2019, 2023) and Health Education England (HEE, 2022) to provide access to clinical work experience in general practice. Effective components of these schemes – typically one week in length – include addressing potential barriers and concerns (e.g., indemnity) by practices (HEE, 2022), sandwiching practical experience between briefing/preparation sessions and post-work experience discussion/reflection sessions, supporting participants to develop their own learning objectives, and providing simple instruments to measure change. This model started in Leeds, spread across Yorkshire, and has since been used as the basis for clinical work experience programmes across the UK (RCGP, 2019). A current estimate is that this type of opportunity is now available to 4–6,000 potential medicine applicants each year in the UK. However, in 2022, there were 24,000 actual applicants and this illustrates one general limitation of outreach – an inability to scale up opportunities to enable all those interested to take part. In this case, accelerated by the Covid-19 pandemic, a number of virtual clinical experience resources have been developed and are generally available (BSMS, 2020; RCGP, 2023), but these may have less impact as they can lack some of the wrap-around elements (e.g., opportunity to ask questions and discuss experiences with doctors, medical students, or other applicants).

Several national initiatives and activities instigated and managed by MSC are discussed in the next section of this chapter.

Widening participation has many regional and local projects; indeed, some of them have spread nationally. One instance is in Lincolnshire, a rural, predominantly agricultural region that set up a Talent Academy in 2016 (Lincolnshire Talent Academy, 2023) that brought together acute hospitals, community trusts, and general practice to address workforce needs by offering programmes to support careers guidance, recruitment, outreach, and clinical work experience.

Focus on national-level actions, initiatives, and coordination

The Alliance was established in 2015, following the SfE final report, to carry out the recommendations therein. Broadly, these fell into three groups of objectives – transparency, equity, and research. Transparency objectives were concerned with the provision of clear and explicit guidance and advice to applicants about how to apply, what medical schools require, and how they select for those requirements. Equity objectives were targeted at the under-represented groups and communities,[5] seeking to counter barriers (perceived and actual) and facilitate application and successful entry to medical school. The research objectives were concerned with producing good evidence about access and participation, fairness of selection criteria and processes, and monitoring the effectiveness of changes to enhance WP. A representative set of Alliance initiatives and activities are described and evaluated below under these three headings.

Equity

The two closely related elements of WP are widening access (getting young people from under-represented communities interested to apply) and selection (devising approaches that improve opportunities for success). Outreach has typically focused on the later years in secondary education, with broad HE activities such as familiarisation with university and advanced-level curriculum support, and medicine-specific outreach, such as taster days (e.g., Leicester Medical School, 2023), summer schools (e.g., Sutton Trust, 2023), and application support (e.g., WAMS Nottingham, 2023), although there are also examples of more longitudinal outreach (e.g., BSMS, 2024).

The Alliance has run a series of summer schools, with funding from Health Education England, since 2016. The approach has been to invite proposals from UK medical schools, commission five, or more, week-long summer schools each year, work with the successful medical schools to agree on programmes, and produce resources that are then shared with the entire sector (MSC, 2023b).

Evaluation of this initiative has run in parallel with the summer schools (Nursaw et al., 2023) and demonstrates a high level of participation with over 1,000 young people having taken part, predominantly from under-represented areas and communities (see Figure 9.4), and discussion of 'cold spots' in the Research section. Reliable and marked increases are evident in participants' self-confidence, communication, understanding of a medical career and the application process, and intention to apply for medicine. Qualitative interviews expanded the understanding of participants' experience. They showed that opportunities to practise elements of the application and selection processes, to meet and talk with doctors and current medical students, and an increasing feeling of safety and self-confidence in the environment were highly valued – all examples of Bandura's theory of self-efficacy (Bandura, 2010; Nursaw et al., 2023). These beneficial outcomes are in line with most published research on the impact of summer schools on access to HE (HEFCE, 2009; Mann and Hoare, 2012; Sharp, 2018).

As with the expansion of clinical work experience, discussed above, one major limitation of summer schools is the number who can participate: perhaps around 1–2,000 per annum if we include all the summer schools run by different universities that contain a medicine strand. Another aspect to consider is the cost per participant that is substantially greater than other forms of outreach (e.g., Evans and Beaney, 2013; Garrud et al., 2018).

Another approach to WP in medicine has been the development of 'Gateway' courses, usually of six years duration (cf. the five-year standard medicine programme). Pioneered by Kings College, London (Garlick and Brown, 2008) in 2001, these courses have WP eligibility criteria (e.g., social and educational disadvantage) and also require lower educational grades.[6] They have been remarkably effective in expanding the number of medical students from under-represented backgrounds (MSC, 2019) although the evidence is mixed about their students' attainment (Curtis and Smith, 2020). At the time of writing, there are 18 gateway courses available, offering roughly 600 places (approximately 6% of medical school places in 2023). These developments have been supported by the Alliance in several ways (e.g., establishing a Gateway/Foundation course forum).

Selection methods in medicine have also changed radically in the 21st century. Admissions tests, for instance, UCAT or GAMSAT, are now routinely used in addition to academic attainment as selection criteria (UCAT, 2023; ACER, 2023), and these are supplemented in most cases by multiple mini-interviews (MMI) – a method that has good evidential support (Terregino et al., 2015; Cleland et al., 2023), and is used to assess personal attributes of candidates. In contrast, hardly any medical schools still use the UCAS personal statement.[7] The Alliance set up an MMI group that has worked with representatives from multiple medical schools, a variety of lay people, and current medical students (from both WP and non-WP backgrounds), supported by expert input from the Work Psychology Group (WPG, 2023), to develop good quality stations (the individual mini-interviews).

After iterative internal review, they are trialed with 1st year medical students and groups of secondary school students before populating a shared MMI station bank that is used by many UK medical schools (MSC, 2019).

The University of Bristol initiated a programme of contextual admissions in 2009 (University of Bristol, 2023) and at the time of publication, offers a two-grade reduction in their standard offer based on A-levels, for applicants: from the 40% most poorly performing schools; from areas of low progression to HE (POLAR 1&2); who have completed a Bristol outreach programme; have a history of being in care or free school meals.

This strategy has resulted in a substantial improvement in the intake of students from disadvantaged backgrounds. In medical schools, adoption of contextual admissions has become a central component in WP, mostly providing reduced offers, and/or a guaranteed interview (e.g., for applicants who have completed an outreach programme). Unfortunately, no national records exist of contextual admissions (e.g., at UCAS or HESA) and so it is difficult to precisely appraise the success of this approach. However, informal indications (personal communication) suggest that medical schools in 2023 admitted between 5% and 40% via a contextual route to their standard entry medicine programmes.

Transparency

An early action was to draw up a uniform specification for every medicine course in the UK and compile these into an annual booklet of entry requirements. This is updated by each medical school and published each year (see: www. medschools.ac.uk/media/3060/uk-medical-school-entry-requirements-202 4-entry.pdf). It has gradually transformed from a paper and electronic booklet into a searchable database plus *pdf* booklet, organised by the four-course types, listing every medicine course in the UK. Feedback from applicants, teachers, and careers advisors has been strongly positive since its inception. It can still develop further, for instance, by providing precise information about the number of places available, application numbers, and performance indicators for successful applicants, such as A-level grades and admission test scores.[8]

Another strand of this work has focused on advice to potential applicants and their advisors (teachers, parents, etc.). This has involved production of short, focused 'Info sheets', booklets for teachers/careers advisors, videos, online webinars, guidance and preparatory materials for interviews, and guidance about work experience, and the core values and attributes needed to study medicine. All these resources, in turn, have been linked together in one website – Studying Healthcare (see: www.medschools.ac.uk/studying-medicine/outreach-and-support/resources-for-teachers-and-students). Web page access counts demonstrate how intensively these resources are used (see Table 9.1).

Research

The success or otherwise of any endeavour to widen access and participation has to be founded on evidence, even if evidence is often partial or lacking initially and arrives later with formal evaluation. SfE identified several crucial evidence gaps and others have become clear over the past decade.

One important source has come from mapping where outreach currently takes place, particularly from medical schools. Starting in 2015, the Alliance has compiled a national outreach map (MSC, 2016, 2018; see Figure 9.4) every two years or so, and this has been used to target new and additional outreach activities at the 'cold spots' – typically geographies and individual schools, or colleges, which have had no engagement with medical schools or,

Table 9.1 Web accesses to key MSC admissions resources

Resource	Monthly average accesses
Entry requirements	15,000
Infosheets	1,000
Work experience	1,600
Teacher/Carer advisor support	1,200

MSC website access

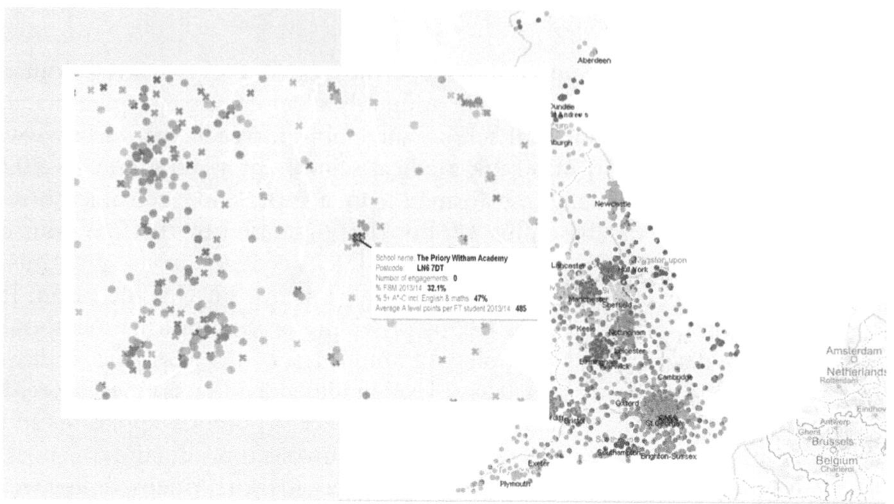

Figure 9.4 MSC 2015 outreach mapping

Source: Top figure shows schools engaged by each medical school; bottom figure gives details from East Midlands (schools engaged with outreach marked by circles, schools not engaged marked by crosses) and an example of a school not receiving outreach in 2015

sometimes, HE at all. Successive mapping exercises, in 2017 and 2019, have shown that outreach has grown and spread in these unengaged areas.

The latest mapping, delayed by the Covid-19 pandemic, is currently under way and, in the interim, other agencies have undertaken similar mapping exercises for outreach (e.g., Laura, 2021; EMWPREP, 2021). Several organisations have commissioned research to expand the evidence base, including The Sutton Trust,[9] Brightside,[10] GMC,[11] and MSC. In 2012, the GMC commissioned a review of medicine admissions (Cleland et al., 2012) that used a combination of literature review and stakeholder interviews to establish the evidence at that time about the validity and equity of selection processes and the effectiveness of widening participation initiatives. This review provided the key groundwork for WP in the following decade. Their main conclusions were that 'no one selection approach is ideal', 'outcome measures used currently to evaluate selection methods focus mostly on medical school attainment rather than being a good doctor', and 'it is clear . . . that the evidence for MMIs, aptitude testing, SJTs and selection centers is better overall than that for traditional interviews, references and autobiographic reports'.

One early piece of MSC-commissioned research explored the impact of changes in admission practices in 18 UK medical schools between 2007 and 2014 (Fielding et al., 2018). The conclusions from this study were that there were no obvious changes in the overall proportion of admissions from each target group, namely, socio-economically disadvantaged, non-selective schools, non-white, and male students. So intractable did changing the medical school demographics appear at that time that the authors advocated radical approaches to selection and a subsequent paper (Cleland et al., 2018) argued that one should think of selection and widening access as 'complex and wicked problems'. This, they argued, may be helpful in foregrounding stakeholder attitudes and context and moving away from the notion of simple interventions. The establishment of five new medical schools in England in 2018 (HEE, 2018) in regions with medical workforce shortages and explicit missions to recruit locally and widen participation was consistent with this proposal, allying universities with established records in widening access and strong local and regional connections with healthcare.

Recognition that data about medicine applicants and entrants, along with information about progression from medical school into postgraduate training was vital, led the GMC, together with MSC and a variety of stakeholders to establish the UK Medical Education Database (UKMED: Dowell et al., 2018; Tang et al., 2022). UKMED has integrated data from multiple sources (e.g., UCAS, HESA, and Royal Colleges) to provide a systematic linkage of information from secondary education qualifications, through admissions metrics, medical school, and both undergraduate and postgraduate outcomes. This resource has enabled a wide variety of research (examples are discussed next) and regular monitoring of trends via public-facing reports (discussed below).

UKMED research (UKMED, 2023) has shown, for instance, that students entering gateway medicine courses complete their qualification in high numbers (>90%), but with lower average attainment scores on the selection metrics for initial postgraduate training (Curtis and Smith, 2020) than comparison groups following standard entry courses at the same medical schools; this attainment deficit also continues into their postgraduate careers (Elmansouri et al., 2023). Another example is work demonstrating the predictive validity of admissions tests (Paton et al., 2022) where performance on UCAT and BMAT, at application to medical school, is positively related to achievement on postgraduate exams. Further examples include a study comparing outcomes for students from state-funded and private (independent) schools (Kumwenda et al., 2017) showing superior attainment, given the same grades at entry, for those from state schools, and one examining the declaration and impact of disability (Murphy et al., 2022) that reported a substantial increase in the proportion of students entering medical school with a disability and comparable success with non-disabled students in completing their course.

Progress in widening access and participation must be monitored in several ways, but one basic requirement is to see how the demographic and socio-economic profile of applicants and entrants to medicine have changed since SfE. The annually updated information held in UKMED provides a direct source of that statistical data and has been used regularly as part of the Alliance's annual reports (e.g., MSC, 2016, 2017, 2018, 2019, 2023a). This monitoring has shown (e.g., the 2019 report) an overall increase in the number of entrants to medical school with demographic characteristics associated with social and economic disadvantage, including the number of entrants from minority ethnic backgrounds (29%, including a 58% increase in students of Black heritage), from the lowest POLAR quintile (35%), from the lowest IMD quintile (46%), from state schools (14%), whose parents do not have HE qualification (11%), and with disabilities (33%). Nevertheless, the absolute numbers are still small in some cases. However, more recent data from this monitoring show that a key target set by SfE to increase the proportion of medicine students from POLAR quintiles 1 and 2 has been met (see Table 9.2). In the subsequent two Covid-19 pandemic years, 2020 and 2021, monitoring has shown no adverse impact on widening access and participation in medicine (Garrud et al., 2023; MSC, 2023a, cf. Eyles et al., 2022).

In addition to the Alliance regular reports, the GMC also has a policy of transparency in producing public reports, about medical education and training, based on extracts of aggregated information from UKMED. Detailed breakdowns of this information can be found on the GMC website (GMC, 2023).

Critical evaluation

As the previous sections of this chapter have documented, the decade since SfE has seen a considerable and sustained effort from the medical school community in widening access and participation. A balanced critique of these efforts, however, must acknowledge that progress, even in terms of the statistics about application and admission profiles, has been limited: compare, for instance, the Scottish Government target of equal progress to HE from every quintile of the Scottish Index of Multiple Deprivation quintile (i.e., 20%, 20%, etc. See Universities Scotland, 2023), with the SfE target (8%, 12%, etc.).

Evaluations of most individual activities have been positive – strong uptake, well received by participants, gains in attitude, skills and career intention, and increased success for targeted under-represented groups – but the degree and scale overall have been restricted. Several of the specific activities are discussed below, but two more general issues will be raised first.

Table 9.2 Proportion of medicine entrants from different POLAR quintiles (1=lowest progression to HE; 5=highest)

POLAR quintile	2013 Actual	2023 target (from SfE report)	2021 Actual
1	5%	8%	9.1%
2	9%	12%	12.8%
3	17%		15.6%
4	23%		20.5%
5	45%		42.1%

Entrants from POLAR quintiles

Virtually all Widening Access and Widening Participation has targeted specific communities, groups, and geographical areas that are under-represented, with the rationale that finite resources are best spent improving the situation of the least advantaged. This has been termed affirmative action since the 1960s in the US, and positive action in the UK, though recently outlawed in America (Supreme Court of the United States, 2023) at least in the form of providing advantages to Black American applicants. Inevitably, targeting can exclude less advantaged individuals who do not quite meet the eligibility criteria (Lambe et al., 2018). Although statistics are lacking to document this effect, it is not an unlikely impact.

There may also be other unintended consequences, including tensions with formerly privileged groups (e.g., Abulafia, 2022), and the stimulation of a commercial industry offering preparation and support for medicine candidates (e.g., McGaghie, 2004; Griffin, 2018) that likely acts as both a real financial and a perceived barrier to disadvantaged potential applicants (Sartania et al., 2021; Lynn, 2023).

Widening access

The mapping exercises have reinforced evidence from SfE (Garrud, 2014; Steven et al., 2016) in showing that there are areas/schools/colleges that are resistant to engagement, despite repeated targeting. This prompts several thoughts: one is to understand the reasons why HE is a low, or non-priority (e.g., a school with low/zero progression to HE, no sixth form, or not providing advanced/higher level science qualifications); another is resourcing (e.g., for careers guidance, though note the Gatsby framework that increased/mandated careers advice (Careers and Enterprise council, 2018)); and a third is to recognise particular challenges of remote and distant locations.

A second issue is the developing recognition that disadvantage is intersectional and not simply a function of minority ethnicity or socio-economic disadvantage. For instance, although access and participation have increased substantially for young people from Black African communities, there has been hardly any improvement for the Black Caribbean community (Garrud et al., 2023; MSC, 2023a). More sophisticated metrics are undoubtedly required to monitor this, such as the UCAS multiple equality measure (UCAS, 2018) and the multidimensional WP measure (Lambe et al., 2018).

The third limitation concerns scale, namely that many outreach activities are difficult if not impossible to scale up to reach every disadvantaged or under-represented community: provision of clinical work experience, discussed earlier, is just one example.

Widening participation

Facilitating entry to medicine for under-represented groups has been the principal rationale for the development of Gateway courses and they are clearly successful in recruiting from those communities (MSC, 2019; Curtis and Smith, 2020). However, the absolute number of places available is still quite limited. In addition, funding an additional year at medical school is a challenge and may deter eligible candidates. There is also an argument (Boliver et al., 2022) that this kind of provision preferentially benefits the less disadvantaged of these groups, a general issue that affects many of the initiatives reviewed in this chapter.

Contextual admissions constitute the other direct mechanism to facilitate entry to medical school, consisting of different or adjusted selection criteria that take account of educational and socio-economic disadvantages. Although contextual admission is now common in medical schools, in many cases it may curtail the opportunities of individuals whose disadvantage (e.g., school attended and parental occupation) does not quite meet the eligibility criteria (sometimes termed the 'squeezed middle', e.g., McCall, 2020). One UK medical school is operating a different form of contextualisation that applies the method to every applicant by assessing their prior educational achievement against the average for their school or college (Chan et al., 2023): it remains to be seen what the broad impact of this radically different approach may be.

Prior educational attainment remains the principal selection criterion and the one directly responsible for under- and over-representation of less and more advantaged groups. There is a long history that justifies this dominant position in selection (e.g., McManus et al., 2013a), even though more recent initiatives, such as admission tests and contextual admissions, have attempted to make adjustments that better identify the ability to succeed at medical school and in medical practice.

Admission tests were introduced in the UK in the early 2000s (GAMSAT in 2001; BMAT in 2003, UCAT/UKCAT in 2006) as an adjunct to secondary educational attainment, primarily to provide a more fine-grained measure of cognitive ability than advanced/higher level grades and degree class. Research since has confirmed a degree of incremental predictive validity (McManus et al., 2013b; Paton et al., 2022), but also demonstrated similar, if less in some respects, sensitivity to disadvantage compared to prior educational attainment (Tiffin et al., 2012, 2014; Cunningham et al., 2023). Some medical schools, in consequence, adjust admission test scores, or apply a lower threshold for WP candidates (e.g., University of Manchester, 2023).

Interviews are usually the second stage in medicine admissions after an initial assessment and shortlisting based on prior academic achievement and admissions test scores. Although, historically, interviews had poor validity and reliability, this has improved with the widespread adoption of multiple mini-interviews (MMIs) – a structured interview that ensures the same challenge to each candidate, trained interviewers who are blind to the candidate's application, and independent judgements spread across a large pool of assessors. Research evidence consistently reports a small advantage overall for female candidates, but, in most cases, a lack of sensitivity to minority ethnicity and other demographic factors (e.g., Knorr et al., 2019; Langer et al., 2020; Sheehan et al., 2023), alongside good reliability and validity (Patterson et al., 2016; Prideaux et al., 2022). It is likely that MMI is a format that does not disadvantage WP candidates, though coaching is becoming more common.

In the last three years, as a response to the Covid-19 pandemic, most interviews have moved to virtual online formats. The MMI format has been successfully transferred, and a variety of novel virtual interview formats have also emerged (e.g., Callwood et al., 2022, 2023). Relatively little formal evaluation has yet been carried out, although informal feedback suggests virtual formats in general are neutral as regards socio-economic disadvantage.

Mentoring, guidance, advice, and coaching

Support for application and admissions has been remarkably successful. An early innovation was the introduction of the Entry Requirements for Medicine annual guide described earlier, where usage has grown substantially each year and it quickly became the principal source of information for applicants and their advisors.

Allied to this have been a wide variety of advice and guidance materials – agreed cross-sector statements about the qualities desired in a doctor, the role of work experience (and the absence of any need for clinical work experience), guidance leaflets and info sheets covering the entire application and selection process for teachers, advisors, and applicants, and a range of video resources (e.g., how to prepare for an MMI) too. This, however, is a contested area with a strong commercial presence as well as a range of alternative free resources, mostly developed by different medical schools (e.g., Future Learn, 2023). For an applicant, the situation remains one where it can be difficult to be sure which offers the best advice, and the commercial resources maintain the perception that it is an advantage to pay for assistance (Eguiguren Wray et al., 2022).

Mentoring, that is having a one-to-one guide with experience and/or expertise in medicine admissions, is highly valued and there is good evidence showing its utility (e.g., Harris and Lane, 2020; Whiting et al., 2020). An Alliance-facilitated scheme that has provided a collaborative mentoring platform with Brightside has been used by several medical schools. Take-up has been good within those universities using Brightside and it is often included as a follow-up component to summer schools and as part of WP access schemes. Nevertheless, young people choose their own mentors when they have the opportunity and so the overall picture is one where many have no access to mentoring, some do (and make good use of it), and others establish relationships with people who may not always have up-to-date information or the relevant expertise and experience.

Next steps

Finally, after critiquing some of the strengths and shortcomings above, it is appropriate to identify some priorities in taking this programme of work forward.

First priorities are to rectify key shortcomings in the original strategy:

- Extending the systematic data monitoring in place (statistical, quantitative) with regular and systematic gathering of evidence about the experience of young people from under-represented communities, who are interested in medicine. This may take the form of regular surveys of experience (e.g., participants in outreach; applicants; and entrants), buttressed by qualitative research (e.g., Rees et al., 2022).
- Building consistent pathways of support, advice, and guidance, that run through from outreach and admissions to success at medical school and into postgraduate training.

The second set of objectives should be concerned with scaling up and extending the outreach and pre-admissions activities. This could include

- Utilising social media to greater effect to engage young people who might consider a career in healthcare – publicising existing resources and promoting opportunities in outreach.
- Continuing to map and analyse 'cold spots' and adopting innovative approaches to engage these schools and colleges.

Lastly, there is value in further evaluation of different selection processes and criteria. A decade has seen strong convergence on 'best practice' in selection (e.g., Cleland et al., 2023), but also the recent establishment of new medical schools and programmes with differentiated missions. Where there is a mandated WP mission, different admissions methods may be better solutions that are transparent and equitable and also aid fulfilment of those undertakings. Examples might be

- Formal comparison of different methods in contextual admissions – 'contextualise everyone' versus target WP applicants.
- Evaluation of synchronous versus asynchronous interviews

Conclusion

In summary, a decade has seen considerable activity in the sector, consistent focus at governmental as well as HE levels, and significant progress in widening access and participation in medicine. Endeavour in the next period should be concerned to extend progress in ways that are more commensurate with the investment and geared to ensure success at medical school and in postgraduate training. As Rainford-Brent (2023) said recently,

> Through all of this pain and reflection the game has gone through, a common question is 'what does progress look like'? It is right to ask. How will we know if we have done a good job, and when? On a basic level, it is representation. If we look at the population, we know roughly how minority communities should be reflected on the field and in the boardroom. It is important to capture the data and hard numbers. More nuanced is charting the experiences of people within the game. It is all very well saying you have invited someone to lunch, but if you then do not make them feel welcome, you have done more harm than good. We need to monitor experiences over time, ask questions and be prepared for honest answers. The same goes for the processes in place for calling out bad experiences. If, in five years, someone needs to call out a problem and feels supported, heard and cared for, then we know the game has progressed.

Notes

1 www.ons.gov.uk/methodology/classificationsandstandards/otherclassifications/ thenationalstatisticssocioeconomicclassificationnssecrebasedonsoc2010   (accessed 22/12/2023). Figure 9.2 depicts the key stakeholders in WP. As can be seen, most organizations were involved, but there were two notable exceptions – the secondary education sector, and prospective medicine students from disadvantaged (WP) backgrounds.
2 In addition to equitable w.r.t. protected characteristics under the UK Equality Act, 2010.
3 Uni Connect: Partnerships set up since 2017 via Office for Students. www.officeforstudents.org.uk/advice-and-guidance/promoting-equal-opportunities/ uni-connect/ (accessed 22/12/2023).
4 NEON: National Education Opportunities Network. www.educationopportunities.co.uk/ (accessed 14/12/2023).
5 Equity of access and participation is both historical and geographical (who is under-represented, when and where); thus, Welsh speakers were poorly represented in the Wales medical schools; communities in coastal areas of England, remote and rural areas of Scotland, and the industrial north-west towns provided few applicants or medical students.
6 Sometimes also combined with local or regional eligibility criteria – for example, a specific London Borough, or Region of England/Scotland/Wales.
7 An autobiographical statement – prone to assistance from others and, occasionally, plagiarism.
8 A growing number of individual medical schools provide some of this information already (e.g., Universities of Manchester www.bmh.manchester.ac.uk/study/ medicine/apply/data/ and Dundee www.dundee.ac.uk/corporate-information/ medicine-admissions-statistics), but a consistent source of information to easily enable potential applicants to compare medicine courses is highly desirable.
9 The Sutton Trust is a social mobility charity. www.suttontrust.com/
10 Brightside – promoting equal opportunities for young people, using mentoring. https://brightside.org.uk/

11 General Medical Council – the professional statutory regulator for medicine. www.
gmc-uk.org/

References

Abulafia, D. (2022, September 1). The truth about getting into Oxbridge. *The Spectator*. www.spectator.co.uk/article/the-truth-about-getting-into-oxbridge/ (accessed 4 December 2023)

ACER. (2023). Graduate medical school admissions test: Assessing capacity to undertake high-level intellectual studies for academic success. *Australian Council for Educational Research*. https://gamsat.acer.org/ (accessed 12 December 2023)

Bandura, A. (2010). Self-Efficacy. In: *The Corsini Encyclopedia of Psychology* (pp. 1–3). American Cancer Society. doi: 10.1002/9780470479216.corpsy0836. ISBN: 978-0-470-47921-6 (accessed 12 December 2023)

BMA. (2023). *Pressures in General Practice Data Analysis.* www.bma.org.uk/advice-and-support/nhs-delivery-and-workforce/pressures/pressures-in-general-practice-data-analysis (accessed 12 December 2023)

Boliver, V., Gorard, S., and Siddiqui, N. (2022). Who counts as socioeconomically disadvantaged for the purposes of widening access to higher education? *British Journal of Sociology of Education*, 43(3), 349–374. doi: 10.1080/01425692.2021.2017852

BSMS. (2020). BSMS virtual work experience. *Brighton and Sussex Medical School.* https://bsmsoutreach.thinkific.com/courses/VWE (accessed 12 December 2023)

BSMS. (2024). BrightMed – Years 9–13 outreach scheme. *Brighton and Sussex Medical School.* www.bsms.ac.uk/about/info-for-schools-teachers-parents/widening-participation-to-medicine.aspx (accessed 15 January 2024)

Callwood, A., Gillam, L., Christidis, A., Doulton, J., Harris, J., Piano, M., Kubacki, A., Tiffin, P. A., Roberts, K., Tarmey, D., and Dalton, D. (2022). Feasibility of an automated interview grounded in Multiple Mini Interview (MMI) methodology for selection into the health professions: An international multimethod evaluation. *BMJ Open*, 12(2), e050394.

Callwood, A., Harris, J., Gillam, L., Roberts, S., Kubacki, A., and Tiffin, P. (2023). Cross-sectional evaluation of an asynchronous Multiple Mini Interview (MMI) in selection to health professions training programmes with ten principles for fairness built-in. *medRxiv*, 2023–03.

Careers & Enterprise Co. (2018). *Understand the Gatsby Benchmarks: A Framework for Best Practice in Careers, and a Key Part of the Government's Careers Strategy.* www.careersandenterprise.co.uk/schools-colleges/understand-gatsby-benchmarks (accessed 29 November 2018)

Chan, P., Anthony, A., Quinlan, K., Smith, S., and Holland, C. (2023). Equity with equality? Contextualising everyone can widen participation in medical school admissions. *Medical Teacher*, 1–8. www.tandfonline.com/doi/abs/10.1080/01421 59X.2023.2287982 (accessed 12 December 2023)

Cleland, J. A., Blitz, J., Cleutjens, K. B., Oude Egbrink, M. G., Schreurs, S., and Patterson, F. (2023). Robust, defensible, and fair: The AMEE guide to selection into medical school: AMEE Guide No. 153. *Medical Teacher*, 1–14.

Cleland, J. A., Dowell, J., McLachlan, J., Nicholson, S., and Patterson, F. (2012). Identifying best practice in the selection of medical students. *GMC Research Report*. www.google.com/search?q=GMC+review+of+medicine+admissions+2012&rlz=1C1GIWA_enGB1053GB1053&oq=GMC+review+of+medicine+admissions+201 2&gs_lcrp=EgZjaHJvbWUyBggAEEUYOTIHCAEQIRigATIHCAIQIRigAdIBC DgzNjhqMGo0qAIAsAIA&sourceid=chrome&ie=UTF-8 (accessed 30 November 2023)

Cleland, J. A., Patterson, F., and Hanson, M. D. (2018). Thinking of selection and widening access as complex and wicked problems. *Medical Education*, 52(12), 1228–1239.

Cunningham, C., Kiezebrink, K., Greatrix, R., Patterson, F., and Vieira, R. (2023). Demographic disparities in dental school selection: An analysis of current UK practices. *European Journal of Dental Education*, 28(1), 56–70.

Curtis, S., and Smith, D. (2020). A comparison of undergraduate outcomes for students from gateway courses and standard entry medicine courses. *BMC Medical Education*, 20, 1–14.

DfES. (2003). *Widening Participation in Higher Education*. https://education-uk.org/documents/pdfs/2003-widening-participation-he.pdf (accessed 22 December 2023)

Dowell, J., Cleland, J., Fitzpatrick, S., McManus, C., Nicholson, S., Oppé, T., Petty-Saphon, K., King, O.S., Smith, D., Thornton, S., and White, K. (2018). The UK Medical Education Database (UKMED) what is it? Why and how might you use it? *BMC Medical Education*, 18, 1–8. doi: 10.1186/s12909-017-1115-9. https://link.springer.com/epdf/10.1186/s12909-017-1115-9?author_access_token=AIOQvS1s72_47ZK1xO9Zpm_BpE1tBhCbnbw3BuzI2RMfrfZmug-MDulEyi9RiB55bHrgLZVMZjiaSNC78Nw7FBOEJcdKRr2g2mHKqXR-wfjAMXuI6v-r-nbmRsaQCZVfvJt9OQOgeqlx-y1cGaSiSRw (accessed 1 December 2023)

Eguiguren Wray, O., Pollard, S. R., and Mountford-Zimdars, A. (2022). An investigation into the contextual admissions information available at UK medical schools' websites: What are the opportunities for enhancement? *Perspectives: Policy and Practice in Higher Education*, 1–10.

Elmansouri, A., Curtis, S., Nursaw, C., and Smith D. (2023). How do the post-graduation outcomes of students from gateway courses compare to those from standard entry medicine courses at the same medical schools? *BMC Medical Education*, 23, 298. doi: 10.1186/s12909-023-04179-3. https://bmcmededuc.biomedcentral.com/articles/10.1186/s12909-023-04179-3 (accessed 1 December 2023)

EMWPREP. (2021). *The National Outreach Coverage Project*. www.emwprep.ac.uk/research/national-outreach-coverage-project/#:~:text=The%20National%20Outreach%20Coverage%20Project,of%20outreach%20delivery%20across%20England (accessed 2 January 2024)

Evans, D. J. R., and Beaney, D. J. (2013). BrightMed: An opportunity to open up anatomy to the next generation. *The FASEB Journal*, 27(S1), 19.4. faseb.onlinelibrary.wiley.com/doi/abs/10.1096/fasebj.27.1_supplement.19.4 (accessed 20 May 2-24)

Eyles, A., Major, L. E., and Machin, S. (2022). *Social Mobility: Past, Present and Future*. London: The Sutton Trust. www.suttontrust.com/our-research/social-mobility-past-present-and-future/ (accessed 7 September 2023)

Fielding, S., Tiffin, P. A., Greatrix, R., et al. (2018). Do changing medical admissions practices in the UK impact on who is admitted? An interrupted time series analysis. *BMJ Open*, 8, e023274. doi: 10.1136/bmjopen-2018-023274

Future Learn. (2023). *Study Medicine: Applying for Medical School and Becoming a Medical Student*. University of Glasgow. www.futurelearn.com/courses/study-medicine (accessed 12 December 2023)

Garlick, P. B., and Brown, G. (2008). Widening participation in medicine. *BMJ*, 336(7653), 1111–1113.

Garrud, P. (2014). Help and hindrance in widening participation; commissioned report. *Medical Schools Council*. www.medschools.ac.uk/media/2446/selecting-for-excellence-research-dr-paul-garrud.pdf (accessed 22 November 2018)

Garrud, P., Hughes, G., Greaves, S., McCracken, S., and Doyle, J. (2018). "I'm a Medic" – A web-based, social capital approach to health careers. *MedEdPublish*, 7(280), 280.

Garrud, P., Wei, Y., and Owen, C. (2023, July). *Impact of the Covid-19 pandemic on UK medical school applications and intake.* ASME Annual Conference, p. 76, Birmingham. www.asme.org.uk/wp-content/uploads/2023/07/Final-Abstracts-Book-2023.pdf (accessed 12 December 2023)

General Medical Council. (2016). *Gateways to the Professions.* www.gmc-uk.org/-/media/documents/Gateways_to_the_professions_Nov_2016.pdf_68375486.pdf (accessed 22 December 2023)

General Medical Council. (2023). *Progression Reports.* https://edt.gmc-uk.org/progression-reports (accessed 1 December 2023)

Griffin, B. (2018). Coaching issues. *Selection and Recruitment in the Healthcare Professions: Research, Theory and Practice,* 223–248.

Harris, P. J., and Lane, K. (2020). Medicine e-mentoring: Accessibility and suitability of e-mentoring for applicants from widening participation and non-widening participation backgrounds. *Widening Participation and Lifelong Learning,* 22(3), 114–136.

Health Education England. (2014). *Widening Participation, It Matters: Our Strategy and Initial Action Plan.* www.hee.nhs.uk/sites/default/files/documents/Widening%20Participation%20it%20Matters_0.pdf (accessed 22 December 2023)

Health Education England. (2018, March 20). *New Medical Schools to Open to Train Doctors of the Future.* www.hee.nhs.uk/news-blogs-events/news/new-medical-schools-open-train-doctors-future (accessed 1 December 2023)

Health Education England. (2022). *Work Experience Resource Toolkits for Health and Care Organisations.* www.hee.nhs.uk/our-work/work-experience-pre-employment-activity/work-experience-resource-toolkits-health-care-organisations (accessed 12 December 2023)

HEPI. (2017). *Where Next for Widening Access and Participation.* www.hepi.ac.uk/wp-content/uploads/2017/08/FINAL-WEB_HEPI-Widening-Participation-Report-98.pdf (accessed 22 December 2023)

Higher Education Funding Council for England. (2009). *Aim Higher Summer Schools Analysis of Provision and Participation 2004 to 2008* [online]. http://webarchive.nationalarchives.gov.uk/20120716090500tf_/www.hefce.ac.uk/pubs/year/2009/200911/ (accessed 28 February 2018)

HMSO. (1997). *The Dearing Report: The Dearing Report (1997) Higher Education in the Learning Society.* London. https://education-uk.org/documents/dearing1997/dearing1997.html (accessed 12 December 2023)

Jeffery, N. (2009, July). Stakeholder engagement: A road map to meaningful engagement (PDF). *The Doughty Centre for Corporate Responsibility, Cranfield School of Management.* Archived from the original (PDF) on 17 April 2015.

Kezar, A. J. (ed.). (2023). *Rethinking Leadership in a Complex, Multicultural, and Global Environment: New Concepts and Models for Higher Education* (1st ed.).New York: Routledge. https://doi.org/10.4324/9781003446842

Knorr, M., et al. (2019). Exploring sociodemographic subgroup differences in Multiple Mini-Interview (MMI) performance based on MMI station type and the implications for the predictive fairness of the Hamburg MMI. *BMC Medical Education,* 19(1), 1–12.

Kumwenda, B., Cleland, J. A., Walker, K., Lee, A. S. J., and Greatrix, R. (2017). The relationship between school type and academic performance at medical school: A national, multi-cohort study. *BMJ Open,* 7, e016291. doi: 10.1136/bmjopen-2017-016291. https://bmjopen.bmj.com/content/7/8/e016291 (accessed 1 December 2023)

Lambe, P., Roberts, M., Gale, T., and Bristow, D. (2018). *UKMED Project P41: Development of a UKMED Multidimensional Measure of Widening Participation Status.* www.ukmed.ac.uk/documents/reports/UKMEDP041_report.pdf (accessed 4 December 2023)

Langer, T., Ruiz, C., Tsai, P., Adams, U., Powierza, C., Vijay, A., Alvarez, P., Dallahan, G. B., and Rahangdale, L. (2020). Transition to multiple mini interview (MMI) interviewing for medical school admissions. *Perspectives on Medical Education*, 9, 229–235.

Laura. (2021). National outreach coverage maps – October 2021. *Tableau Public*. https://public.tableau.com/app/profile/laura8331/viz/GradientandSpotMapforAA-WithMapLayerViews-CoverageSept2021/OutreachActivities201718–201920 (accessed 30 November 2023)

Leicester Medical School. (2023). *Outreach*. https://le.ac.uk/medicine/outreach (accessed 12 December 2023)

Lincolnshire Talent Academy. (2023). https://lincstalentacademy.org.uk/ (accessed 6 September 2023)

Lynn, E. (2023). Widening participation is for life, not just for admissions. *BMJ*, 383, 2659 www.bmj.com/content/383/bmj.p2659 (accessed 4 December 2023)

Mann, R. and Hoare, T. (2012). *The Impact of the Sutton Trust's Summer Schools on Subsequent Higher Education Participation: A Report to the Sutton Trust* [online]. https://www.suttontrust.com/our-research/impact-sutton-trusts-summer-schools-subsequent-higher-education-participation-report-sutton-trust/ (accessed 20 May 2024)

McCall, A. (2020, February 2). University reform is the squeezed middle's new worry: A drive to get top institutions to accept disadvantaged pupils may have unintended consequences. *The Times*, London. www.thetimes.co.uk/article/university-reform-is-the-squeezed-middles-new-worry-g9t00d3rs (accessed 12 December 2023)

McGaghie, W. C., Downing, S. M., and Kubilius, R. (2004). What is the impact of commercial test preparation courses on medical examination performance? *Teaching and Learning in Medicine*, 16(2), 202–211. doi: 10.1207/s15328015tlm1602_14

McManus, I. C., Dewberry, C., Nicholson, S., and Dowell, J. S. (2013b). The UKCAT-12 study: Educational attainment, aptitude test performance, demographic and socio-economic contextual factors as predictors of first year outcome in a cross-sectional collaborative study of 12 UK medical schools. *BMC Medicine*, 11, 1–25.

McManus, I. C., Woolf, K., Dacre, J., Paice, E., and Dewberry, C. (2013a). The academic backbone: Longitudinal continuities in educational achievement from secondary school and medical school to MRCP (UK) and the specialist register in UK medical students and doctors. *BMC Medicine*, 11(1), 1–27.

Medical Schools Council. (2016). *Implementing Selecting for Excellence a Progress Update*. www.medschools.ac.uk/media/1207/selecting-for-excellence-2016-update-msc.pdf (accessed 12 December 2023)

Medical Schools Council. (2017). *Selection Alliance 2017 Report an Update on the Medical Schools Council's Work in Selection and Widening Participation*. www.medschools.ac.uk/media/2388/msc-selection-alliance-2017-report.pdf (accessed 12 December 2023)

Medical Schools Council. (2018). *Selection Alliance 2018 Report an Update on the Medical Schools Council's Work in Selection and Widening Participation*. www.medschools.ac.uk/media/2536/selection-alliance-2018-report.pdf (accessed 12 December 2023)

Medical Schools Council. (2019). *Selection Alliance 2019 Report an Update on the Medical Schools Council's Work in Selection and Widening Participation*. www.medschools.ac.uk/media/2608/selection-alliance-2019-report.pdf (accessed 12 December 2023)

Medical Schools Council. (2023a). *MSC Selection Alliance Annual Report 2023: An Update on the Medical Schools Council's Work in Selection and Widening Participation*. www.medschools.ac.uk/media/3125/selection-alliance-update-2023.pdf (accessed 20 May 2024)

Medical Schools Council. (2023b). *MSC Summer Schools*. www.medschools.ac.uk/our-work/selection/msc-summer-schools (accessed 12 December 2023)

Milburn, A. (2012). Fair access to professional careers. *The Independent Reviewer on Social Mobility and Child Poverty*. https://assets.publishing.service.gov.uk/media/5a78a420e5274a277e68e514/IR_FairAccess_acc2.pdf (accessed 22 December 2023)

MSC. (2014). *Selecting for Excellence: Final Report*. www.medschools.ac.uk/media/1203/selecting-for-excellence-final-report.pdf (accessed 12 December 2023)

Murphy, M. J., Dowell, J. S., and Smith, D. T. (2022). Factors associated with declaration of disability in medical students and junior doctors, and the association of declared disability with academic performance: Observational study using data from the UK Medical Education Database, 2002–2018 (UKMED54). *BMJ Open*, 12, e059179. doi: 10.1136/bmjopen-2021-059179. https://bmjopen.bmj.com/content/12/4/e059179 (accessed 1 December 2023)

Nicholls, G., Blythe, A., and Pearson, D. (2012). Making an educational case for a national primary care curriculum for medical students: Lessons from one UK medical school. *Education for Primary Care*, 23(5), 313–316.

Nursaw, C., Garrud, P., Owen, C., Jackson, D., and Wei, Y. (2023, July). *Diversifying medicine*. ASME Annual Conference, p. 76, Birmingham. www.asme.org.uk/wp-content/uploads/2023/07/Final-Abstracts-Book-2023.pdf (accessed 12 December 2023)

Office for Students. (2023). *Medical and Dental Students Survey 2023*. www.officeforstudents.org.uk/advice-and-guidance/funding-for-providers/health-education-funding/medical-and-dental-intakes/ (accessed 12 December 2023)

Patterson, F., Knight, A., Dowell, J., Nicholson, S., Cousans, F., and Cleland, J. (2016). How effective are selection methods in medical education? A systematic review. *Medical Education*, 50(1), 36–60.

Paton, L. W., McManus, I. C., Cheung, K. Y. F., Smith, D. T., and Tiffin, P. A. (2022). Can achievement at medical admission tests predict future performance in postgraduate clinical assessments? A UK-based national cohort study. *BMJ Open*, 12, e056129. doi: 10.1136/bmjopen-2021-056129. https://bmjopen.bmj.com/content/12/2/e056129 (accessed 1 December 2023)

Prideaux, D., Roberts, C., Eva, K., Centeno, A., McCrorie, P., McManus, C., Patterson, F., Powis, D., Tekian, A., and Wilkinson, D. (2022). Assessment for selection for the health care professions and specialty training. In: *International Best Practices for Evaluation in the Health Professions* (pp. 77–96). London: CRC Press.

Rainford-Brent, E. (2023). *ICEC Report: Ebony Rainford-Brent Says Cricket Can become UK's Most Inclusive Sport*. www.bbc.co.uk/sport/cricket/66902424

RCGP. (2019). Widening participation work experience programme. *Royal College of General Practitioners*. London. www.rcgp.org.uk/getmedia/97df16db-c0d4-4d48-9514-c23f6a6efbe4/RCGP-WP-Work-Experience-overview-October-2019.pdf (accessed 12 December 2023)

RCGP. (2023). Observe GP. *Royal College of General Practitioners*. London. www.rcgp.org.uk/your-career/work-experience/observe-gp (accessed 12 December 2023)

Rees, E. L., Mattick, K., Harrison, D., Rich, A., and Woolf, K. (2022). "I'd have to fight for my life there": A multicentre qualitative interview study of how socioeconomic background influences medical school choice. *Medical Education Online*, 27(1), 2118121.

Robinson, D., and Salvestrini, V. (2020). The impact of interventions for widening access to higher education: A review of the evidence. *Education Policy Institute*. https://epi.org.uk/publicationsand-research/impact-of-interventions-for-widening-access-to-he (accessed 22 December 2023)

Sartania, N., Alldridge, L., and Ray, C. (2021). Barriers to access, transition and progression of Widening Participation students in UK medical schools: The students' perspective. *MedEdPublish*, 10, 132. doi: 10.15694/mep.2021.000132.1

Schwartz, S. (2004). Fair admissions to higher education: Recommendations for good practice. *London: Higher Education Steering Group.* https://dera.ioe.ac.uk/id/eprint/5284/1/finalreport.pdf (accessed 22 December 2023)

Scottish Funding Council. (2005). *Learning for All: The Report of the SFEFC/SHEFC Widening Participation Review Group.* http://archive.sfc.ac.uk/publications/pubs_other_sfcarchive/learning_for_all_publication_september_2005.pdf (accessed 29 January 2010)

Sharp, C. (2018). Can summer schools improve outcomes for disadvantaged pupils? NFER social mobility briefing. *National Foundation for Educational Research.* http://files.eric.ed.gov/fulltext/ED590446.pdf (accessed 7 September 2023)

Sheehan, A., Thomson, R., Arundell, F., and Pierce, H. (2023). A mixed methods evaluation of multiple mini interviews for entry into the bachelor of midwifery. *Women and Birth*, 36(2), 193–204.

Social Mobility and Child Poverty Commission. (2014). Elitist Britain. *London: Social Mobility and Child Poverty Commission.*

Social Mobility Commission. (2016). *Social Mobility and the Professions.* https://assets.publishing.service.gov.uk/media/5a75b9a240f0b67f59fcf202/The_Professions_factsheet.pdf (accessed 22 December 2023)

Steven, K., Dowell, J., Jackson, C., and Guthrie, B. (2016). Fair access to medicine? Retrospective analysis of UK medical schools application data 2009–2012 using three measures of socioeconomic status. *BMC Medical Education*, 16, 1–10.

Supreme Court of the United States. (2023) Students for Fair Admissions, Inc. v. President and Fellows of Harvard College. Certiorari to the United States Court of Appeals for the first circuit No. 20–1199. Argued October 31, 2022—Decided June 29, 2023. www.supremecourt.gov/opinions/22pdf/20-1199_hgdj.pdf (accessed 29 June 2023).

The Sutton Trust. (2023). *Pathways to Medicine.* https://pathwaysprogrammes.suttontrust.com/career-pathways/medicine (accessed 12 December 2023)

Tang, P., Sierocinska-King, O., Petty-Saphon, K., Smith, D., Oppé, T., Thornton, S., and Dowell, J. (2022). Where graduates go? A case study of the United Kingdom Medical Education Database (UKMED). In: *Strengthening the Collection, Analysis and Use of Health Workforce Data and Information: A Handbook* (Ch. 5). Geneva: World Health Organisation. www.who.int/publications/i/item/9789240058712

Terregino, C. A., McConnell, M., and Reiter, H. I. (2015). The effect of differential weighting of academics, experiences, and competencies measured by Multiple Mini Interview (MMI) on race and ethnicity of cohorts accepted to one medical school. *Academic Medicine*, 90(12), 1651–1657.

Tiffin, P. A., Dowell, J. S., and McLachlan, J. C. (2012). Widening access to UK medical education for under-represented socioeconomic groups: Modelling the impact of the UKCAT in the 2009 cohort. *BMJ*, 344.

Tiffin, P. A., McLachlan, J. C., Webster, L., and Nicholson, S. (2014). Comparison of the sensitivity of the UKCAT and A Levels to sociodemographic characteristics: A national study. *BMC Medical Education*, 14(1), 1–12.

UCAS. (2018). *MEM Summary Report.* www.ucas.com/file/190246/download?token=7drEUmCm (accessed 4 December 2023)

UCAT Consortium. (2023). *About the University Clinical Aptitude Test (UCAT).* www.ucat.ac.uk/#:~:text=The%20University%20Clinical%20Aptitude%20Test%20(UCAT)%20is%20an%20admissions%20test,UCAS%20application%20and%20academic%20qualifications. (accessed 12 December 2023)

UKMED. (2023). *Published Research.* www.ukmed.ac.uk/published_research (accessed 1 December 2023)

Universities Scotland. (2023). *Widening Access to Medicine.* www.universities-scotland. ac.uk/bite-size-briefings/widening-access-to-medicine/ (accessed 2 September 2023)

University of Bristol. (2023). *Our Position On: Contextual University Offers.* www.bristol.ac.uk/media-library/sites/policybristol/position-papers/UOB%20Position%20 Paper%20Contextual%20Offers%202023.pdf (accessed 20 May 2024)

University of Manchester. (2023). *Widening Participation Programmes for Medicine Courses.* www.bmh.manchester.ac.uk/study/medicine/apply/widening-access/ widening-participation-programmes/ (accessed 6 December 2022)

WAMS Nottingham. (2023). *Widening Access to Medicine.* www.facebook.com/WAMSNottingham/ (accessed 12 December 2023)

Whiting, J. R., Wickham, S., and Beaney, D. (2020). Medical student mentors in widening access to medicine programmes: "We're lighting fires, not filling buckets". *Widening Participation and Lifelong Learning*, 22(2), 205–224.

Work Psychology Group. (2023). www.workpsychologygroup.com/case-study/high-stakes-assessment-in-healthcare/ (accessed 9 September 2023)

Chapter 10

Doctors in schools

Breaking down barriers to the profession

*Anjali Vaidyanathan, Enam Haque,
and Albert Jennings*

Introduction

In the United Kingdom (UK), Medicine has traditionally been seen as a career for the elite or privileged in society, with students from low socio-economic backgrounds remaining under-represented in medical education (Gore et al., 2018). Despite efforts to increase gender parity and ethnic diversity among UK doctors, the lack of people from lower socio-economic backgrounds entering the profession is unfortunately still the reality (BMA, 2023). This is hugely detrimental, not only to the talented students who feel that applying to Medicine is out of their reach but also to patients and society. Professional bodies such as the British Medical Association (BMA) have recognised the importance of encouraging those with the relevant academic potential to regard medicine as a viable option, irrespective of their socio-economic circumstances (BMA, 2023). The Medical Schools Council (MSC) have recently published a report emphasising the need to expand medical school places to meet increasing workforce demands in the NHS (National Health Service) (Medical Schools Council, 2021). Moreover, they have stressed the importance of using a wider talent pool to achieve these aims, with widening participation being at the heart of this. We therefore recognise the need for immediate initiatives to be implemented to move this mission forward.

The importance of role modelling – Dr Enam Haque

Role modelling is defined as 'a person who someone admires and whose behaviour they try to copy' (Cambridge Dictionary, 2023). Why is role modelling important in widening participation? In an online survey of medical students by Sartania et al. (2021), students stated that there were three key perceived barriers to successful admission to medical school, in line with Bourdieu's different forms of capital; this was reduced/different economic, social, and cultural capital compared to their peers. In terms of social capital, they felt that they lacked the necessary connections among family and friends to obtain relevant work experience or insight into a medical career. Their cultural capital did not match to admissions interviewers' cultural capital, and so they were less likely to be successful in the process.

DOI: 10.4324/9781003399858-10

Looking at drivers for WP pupils to apply to medical school, McHarg et al. (2007) noted the importance that role models played for aspiring medical students from this background. They suggested that medical schools needed to build aspirations in their outreach work, emphasising the importance of selecting role models that were medical students from diverse backgrounds.

Doctors can also be effective role models. Passi et al. (2013) conducted a systematic review, looking at the impact of doctors as role models in medical education. They found that they helped to influence career decisions for both medical students and postgraduate trainees. This was through actively engaging students while on clinical placements or showing a passion for their career choice. These qualities could be emulated for medical students attending a work experience placement or listening to a talk by an inspiring doctor. One method to provide role modelling for WP pupils is through structured mentoring. Smith et al. (2013) described an e-mentoring programme they offered to WP pupils in London. Pupils were assigned to a medical student mentor and online communication was through a secure website, managed by the charity, Brightside Trust. In total, 147 pupils completed the e-mentoring scheme over three years, with the mentoring lasting six months, on average. Unfortunately, the study could not trace the outcomes for most Year 12 pupils who took part in the e-mentoring.

Mentoring can also take place in person. Whiting et al. (2020) looked at a mentoring initiative run by Brighton and Sussex Medical School. Using focus groups to explore the experience of medical student mentors, they noted key qualities that enabled effective mentoring. These included being friendly, confident, and approachable, as well as sharing their experiences of life at medical school. Although mentors felt they needed to understand the background of their mentees, they did not feel they necessarily had to come from the same background. Their perception was that the key aspects of being a mentor were offering pastoral support and building a strong relationship with their mentee.

Role modelling can also be undertaken through delivering talks to aspiring medical students. Sanders et al. (2018) conducted a randomised control trial looking at the impact of inspirational talks, covering life in university, by University of Bristol students. They found the intervention significantly and positively impacted on successful applications to university. The University of Manchester Medical School has followed a similar programme, but with doctors providing the inspirational talks. The aim is to challenge the 'privileged knowledge of the system', whereby pupils with friends and relatives in medical careers can gain invaluable insight into becoming a doctor (Sartania et al., 2021). This is a luxury that those from widening participation backgrounds do not have access to.

Case study: doctors as 'widening participation champions' in schools

WP in higher education has been a hallmark of the University of Manchester's vision; enabling fairer access to higher education for talented students from all backgrounds has been central to the University's values as a world-class university (University of Manchester, 2023a). Central to this vision are WP programmes and activities to level this playing field and enable less privileged yet talented pupils to access Medical Degrees (Salam, 2010). This will then promote a diverse medical profession and ensure selection of future doctors is from a wide meritocratic student pool. This diversity has been shown to provide healthcare benefits and promote social mobility (Girotti et al., 2015; Hayton and Paczusk, 2003; Magnus and Mick, 2000). In keeping with our institution's values and vision, we are motivated in ensuring less-privileged pupils have the chance to enter medical school (University of Manchester, 2023b) and are committed to developing innovative programmes of activity in this area.

The medical school WP team recognised a specific need to establish outreach in secondary schools in 2015, and as a result established the 'Doctors in Schools' initiative. This outreach activity is aimed at local secondary schools in Greater Manchester that meet specific criteria. It involves the WP team sending doctors into schools to deliver talks and other educational activities to inspire pupils and help to dispel perceived myths.

The criteria for the schools selected are based around algorithms set to target schools that need the most support. The key criteria are that of

- Lower income families/those deemed to be in low socio-economic groups.
- Postcodes where Higher Education participation is low.
- First generation to enter Higher Education.
- Schools and colleges where performance is below the national average.
- Disability
- Caring responsibilities
- Ethnic under-representation

Through this, we have been able to curate a database of local schools that we feel are in the most need. We have developed positive working relationships with teachers and staff in these schools. Staff members can directly contact the team if they wish to have a talk on medicine for their pupils. There are now 15–20 schools in the Greater Manchester area which regularly request talks from the 'Doctors in Schools' team, and we plan to expand this number over the coming years.

The content of the Doctors in Schools sessions is based around the needs of the school and can be adapted to specific requirements. For that reason, we remain very flexible in our approach. Sometimes, schools want a talk on a specific topic (for example, 'A Day in the Life of a GP'), or to commemorate a particular calendar event (for example, National STEMM week or International Women's Day); whereas at other times the school may simply want a doctor from a similar background to come in and give a brief presentation about their journey into Medicine. Overall, the theme and content can be fluid and led by the doctor attending.

Due to variation in the types of sessions that different schools may require, we have developed a bespoke training package for doctors wanting to take on this work. This is to help guide them and give them tips and tricks on the differing activity they may be involved in. Recruitment of doctors is on an expression of interest basis (for example, doctors who have approached us about their interest in widening participation), as well as advertising our training sessions to local GPs and hospital doctors through our links with the teaching hospitals and practices. The doctors who enrol for the training can be from any speciality and at any point in their career, from Foundation trainees, to post Completion of Certificate of Training (CCT) consultants and GPs. This is to promote and encourage a wide pool of doctors into this work, from all ages and levels of training. Once they have attended the training, the doctors officially become 'Widening Participation Champions' for the University of Manchester. A key point to note is that the doctors do not need to be from a widening participation background themselves to engage in this work. This role is a key responsibility as per the GMC guidance for all medics to demonstrate commitment to social responsibility (GMC, 2022) and promote collaboration with local communities.

The CPD-accredited training session is called 'Becoming a Widening Participation Champion' and is held face to face in the University campus. It is recognised as a University of Manchester Medical School PRIME (Professionals in Medical Education) staff development training session and comprises various segments to meet the learning objectives required to enable them to engage in this work. We cover areas including:

- A background to Widening Participation
- Discussions around why it is important
- Brief overview of the MB ChB requirements, the UCAT exam, and interview/admissions processes
- Practical tips and ideas for workshops and presentations
- The 'Doctors in Schools' events – what we have done already, upcoming events, feedback, next steps in how they get involved

We have established close links with the medical admissions team, to ensure that all admissions-related information is up to date. This ensures that any messages related to applying to the University of Manchester are factually correct.

All training sessions are quality-assured using written evaluation questionnaires. For our most recent session in 2023, the evaluation was extremely positive, with 100% of attendees stating that they felt the session would 'prepare them well' to participate in Doctors in Schools events.

Once a secondary school has contacted us for a WP Champion to attend, we send an email to our bank of trained Widening Participation Champions. The session is allocated on a first come first served basis and there is no minimum or maximum number of sessions that a WP Champion undertakes. We actively encourage more than one doctor to attend each event, if feasible (and if the school is happy with this), as this demonstrates the varied nature of the work and roles of doctors. This also instils camaraderie and offers an opportunity to network with a colleague within the Champions group. The selected Champion(s) will then liaise directly with the teacher at the school to confirm the finer details of the event and the logistics. Given the altruistic nature of this work (there is no remuneration for the doctors attending the schools), the schools are encouraged to be flexible and accommodating to the needs of the Champions, and we work with all parties to ensure the smooth running and planning of the events.

In the past year, we have successfully delivered six school events. The feedback we have received has been immensely positive from both the Champions attending, and the schools themselves. School feedback is through the lead teacher, based on their own thoughts and a collation of the pupils' feedback. All of the schools we engaged scored 5/5 for satisfaction, and 100% stated 'very much so' to the question 'Do you feel this event may now help inspire your pupils into a career in Medicine?' This demonstrates the immense benefit of our programme, which we hope will then translate into motivated pupils exploring medicine as a career option.

Doctors in Schools doesn't come without its challenges. As mentioned earlier, the WP Champions are practising clinicians who give up their spare time for the outreach work. The schools normally prefer a Champion to attend during school hours, which may be during their clinical hours. In addition, as there is no remuneration for the work, there is reduced incentive for them to prioritise this over paid work. The role does not offer the benefits that University of Manchester staff receive, including access to facilities and resources. With the lack of monetary benefit, it does rely on the willingness of Champions to give up their spare time.

So, what next? Given the successes we have achieved so far, we plan to expand our Doctors in Schools programme. We have widened our 'bank' of Champions and have increased the numbers of schools we work with. From an MB ChB programme level, our next aim is to involve medical students in the Doctors in Schools events, incorporating ideals of 'Service-Learning' and student-led presentations. The benefit of service learning is that it 'appears to provide simultaneous opportunities to train students authentically, engage the community and university reciprocally, and develop students' cognitive-emotional dimensions' (Stewart and Wubbena, 2014). The students would attend alongside the Champions and offer a closer near-peer level of inspiration to the pupils, whilst also improving the students' own confidence in communicating.

On a national scale, we are aiming to collaborate with other UK Medical Schools. We recently delivered a presentation at the National Medical Schools Widening Participation Forum Conference in 2023. We also presented our work at the Association for the Study of Medical Education (ASME) Annual Conference in July 2023, whose theme was around creating a diverse workforce. The presentations enabled us to highlight our work, share best practice, and demonstrate the successful reach and importance of this programme.

References

BMA. (2023). *Widening Participation in Medicine*. www.bma.org.uk/advice-and-support/studying-medicine/becoming-a-doctor/widening-participation-in-medicine (accessed 6 December 2023)

Cambridge Dictionary ROLE MODEL | English Meaning-Cambridge Dictionary (accessed 6 December 2023)

General Medical Council. (2022). *Corporate Social Responsibility (CSR)-GMC*. gmc-uk.org (accessed 6 December 2023)

Girotti, J. A., Park, Y. S., and Tekian, A. (2015). Ensuring a fair and equitable selection of students to serve society's health care needs. *Medical Education*, 49, 84–92. doi: 10.1111/medu.12506

Gore, J., Patfield, S., Holmes, K., and Smith, M. (2018). Widening participation in medicine? New insights from school students' aspirations. *Medical Education*, 52(2), 227–238. doi: 10.1111/medu.13480

Hayton, A., and Paczusk, A. (2003). Introduction: Education in demand? In: *Access, Participation and Higher Education* (1st ed.). Policy & Practice. Abingdon, UK: Routledge.

Magnus, S. A., and Mick, S. S. (2000). Medical schools, affirmative action, and the neglected role of social class. *American Journal of Public Health*, 90(8), 1197–1201. doi: 10.2105/ajph.90.8.1197. PMID: 10936995; PMCID: PMC1446350.

McHarg, J., Mattick, K., and Knight, L. V. (2007). Why people apply to medical school: Implications for widening participation activities. *Medical Education*, 41, 815–821. doi: 10.1111/j.1365-2923.2007.02798.x

Medical Schools Council. (2021). www.medschools.ac.uk/news/medical-schools-call-for-increase-in-doctors-to-support-nhs-recovery-and-sustainability (accessed 6 December 2023)

Passi, V., Johnson, S., Ed Peile, Wright, S., Hafferty, F., and Johnson, N. (2013). Doctor role modelling in medical education: BEME Guide No. 27. *Medical Teacher*, 35(9), e1422–e1436. doi: 10.3109/0142159X.2013.806982

Salam, A. (2010). Widening participation. *BMJ*, 340, c108. doi: 10.1136/bmj.c108

Sanders, M., Burgess, S., Chande, R., Dilnot, C., Kozman, E., and Macmillan, L. (2018). Role models, mentoring and university applications-evidence from a crossover randomised controlled trial in the United Kingdom. *Widening Participation and Lifelong Learning*, 20(4), 57–80.

Sartania, N., Alldridge, L., and Ray, C. (2021). Barriers to access, transition, and progression of Widening Participation students in UK medical schools: The students' perspective [version 1]. *MedEdPublish*, 10, 132. doi: 10.15694/mep.2021.000132.1

Smith, S., Alexander, A., Dubb, S., Murphy, K., and Laycock, J. (2013). Opening doors and minds: A path for widening access. *The Clinical Teacher*, 10, 124–128. doi: 10.1111/j.1743-498X.2012.00616.x

Stewart, T., and Wubbena, Z. (2014). An overview of infusing service-learning in medical education. *International Journal of Medical Education*, 5, 147–156. doi: 10.5116/ijme.53ae.c907. PMID: 25341224; PMCID: PMC4212253.

University of Manchester. (2023a). *Widening Participation in Higher Education*. www.manchester.ac.uk/connect/teachers/students/widening-participation/ (accessed 6 December 2023)

University of Manchester. (2023b). *Widening Participation Programmes for Medicine Courses*. www.bmh.manchester.ac.uk/study/medicine/apply/widening-access/widening-participation-programmes/ (accessed 6 December 2023)

Whiting, J. R., Wickham, S., and Beaney, D. (2020). Medical student mentors in widening access to medicine programmes: "We're lighting fires, not filling buckets". *Widening Participation and Lifelong Learning*, 22(20), 205–224.

Chapter 11

Supporting (early) professional development for students from widening participation backgrounds

Sally Curtis, Jacquie Kelly, and Chloe Langford

The impact of the WP context and the need for support

Introduction

For WP students, medical schools offer contextual admissions and gateway courses as routes into medical school, both of which offer grade reductions from the normal entry requirements.

Many WP students thrive at medical school requiring minimal support, despite a high number coming from families without experience of Higher Education (HE) or professional backgrounds (Curtis and Smith, 2020). However, such backgrounds can also impede the development of a professional identity and reduce feelings of belonging (Mathers and Parry, 2009).

Research shows that WP students, students from other under-represented backgrounds and students with intersected identities can lack a sense of belonging and feel marginalised for a variety of reasons (Frost and Regehr, 2013). These include a lack of understanding from staff and other students, feelings of imposter syndrome, financial difficulties, and the challenges of undertaking paid employment while studying, and a 'white-centric', often classed curriculum with a lack of diversity in clinical examples, resources, staff, and sim patients (Bunce et al., 2019; Canning et al., 2020; Friedman, 2014; Elliott et al., 2013; Verbree et al., 2023).

Policies and learning environments within medical schools and clinical training are also associated with poorer academic outcomes for students from ethnic minorities compared to white students (Woolf et al., 2011; Nazar et al., 2015), and, recently, there has been an increase in awareness of the need to diversify the curriculum to be representative of the population and to support safe and inclusive medical education for students (MSC, 2021). There is now greater acknowledgement of the impact of the learning environment and curriculum on students' sense of belonging and inclusion at medical school, including the need for representative diversity in sim patients, anatomical models, and case studies in the curriculum.

DOI: 10.4324/9781003399858-11

Evaluation of the progression of WP students has shown that attrition rates are often higher and there is an awarding gap (also referred to as the attainment gap or differential attainment) both on entry and exit from medical school. However, comparing WP student performance with their traditional entry peers, who do not share similar challenges, does not always provide a representative picture of their achievements, which can feed into an unhelpful student deficit discourse. This deficit discourse presents these students as being the root of the problem because of their own inadequacies or characteristics and implies that students must solve their problems for them to succeed academically (McKay and Devlin, 2016). Additionally, there is no acknowledgement of the institutional barriers in place that can cause many of the problems students face. This discourse can contribute to marginalisation, ultimately resulting in or compounding experiences of alienation and a lack of belonging and self-confidence.

Having overcome hurdles to access higher education, successful completion of the course often requires students from low socio-economic backgrounds to adapt to an unfamiliar social environment (Reay et al., 2009). In a study examining the costs of seeking upward social mobility for working-class students at elite universities (Jetten et al., 2008), authors suggested that the mismatch in social identity between attending a high-status university and coming from a low-status background created tension and unease and was often a price that can be too high to pay. Where the university environment was aligned to students' social background, the transition appeared relatively smooth, but students from communities with a very different culture faced a greater challenge to their social identity and risked losing connections with their family and friends. In navigating the disparity between their past and present identity, students may choose to be open about their background or prefer to be guarded about it, or even imitate an alternative identity to avoid anticipated stigma (Warner et al., 2007).

Individuals who have less cultural awareness of higher education may misinterpret this inexperience as lack of ability; this is particularly common among those experiencing Impostor Syndrome (Rakestraw, 2017). While Impostor Syndrome is generally viewed as affecting those who feel that they lack competence in a subject or skill, it has also been shown to impact students from under-represented backgrounds, who may believe that their race, ethnicity, or social class are the reason they do not belong in a given environment. Students who feel this way may then be more prone to perceive feedback as a personal indictment, regardless of its intent. This makes it even more vital that staff and peers are aware of their own potential biases and respect all students' contributions and backgrounds.

Entering medical school is a key transition point, as is the progression to full-time clinical placements, and these transition points have emerged as risk factors for WP student attrition. Researchers reported that building relationships and supportive interventions to support progression at such times can overcome this (Cotton et al., 2017; Caruana et al., 2011). The financial cost of studying may also impact student attrition (Department for Education, 2019). Anane and Curtis (2022) reported that students from low socio-economic backgrounds had no choice but to undertake paid employment and had to prioritise survival over their studies, compared to their more affluent peers who could choose when to work and prioritise their education when required. Providing additional financial support, for example, in the form of bursaries, may help to alleviate some of the challenges which are typically faced by students from lower socio-economic backgrounds that contribute to attrition (Harrison and Hatt, 2012; Hatt et al., 2003). However, financial inducements are reported to be less effective for student retention than feeling socially comfortable at the institution (Harrison and Hatt, 2012).

Universities have an obligation to provide appropriate support to enable students to develop self-confidence and a sense of professional identity. Although they cannot mitigate all the factors mentioned in this section, they can improve the experience for WP students with a better understanding of the challenges that students face and acknowledging their responsibility within those challenges. The following interventions can be employed to help WP medical students develop their sense of professional identity and support them during key points of transition.

Early healthcare or community placements

The social networks of many students from WP backgrounds do not provide access to work experience opportunities often afforded to those from more advantaged and professional family backgrounds. This disparity has been recognised through updated national guidance for applicants (MSC, 2020) and accommodated through medical schools' admissions processes, with only a few requiring work experience from applicants. Although work experience is still welcomed, it is acknowledged that life experiences also provide rich and relevant opportunities for reflection and personal learning that can demonstrate motivation and insight into what is required of a medical student.

Whilst work experience in a healthcare setting is not now required for most medical school applications, it can be an important factor in determining whether medicine is the right career choice and the first step in grounding students' ambition to become a doctor in real-world experience. For students who have not previously experienced healthcare settings, placements and community engagement can provide an opportunity to consolidate their motivation to study medicine and begin the process of identity formation as a healthcare professional.

Embedding placements within a professionalism module from the start of their course ensures WP students have experience of a variety of healthcare environments and of the NHS as an organisation. Placements introduce early patient contact and provide insight into the variety of roles within the NHS and can support the development of communication skills with both patients and staff in professional environments. Alternating placements with classroom-based sessions can also consolidate theoretical learning, especially in subjects such as sociology and psychology as applied to medicine and public health, which can be readily applied across different settings. Placements also provide access to role models, and framing these experiences within a professionalism module supports professional identity development for WP students by situating their experiences in the context of what it is to be a medical professional.

Classroom sessions can be structured to help students prepare for and reflect on their experiences in the clinical setting and identify their own learning and professional development. These sessions can also enhance social networks of support, particularly when students lack a sense of belonging, as they may not realise others share similar thoughts and feelings to themselves. Discussion groups or group reflections held after attending placements have been shown to provide safe spaces for students to share concerns or questions and can normalise experiences, thoughts, and feelings, and providing opportunities to share openly can facilitate and legitimise their sense of belonging and shared professional identity.

Working with identity and inclusivity

WP medical students have a diverse range of backgrounds and experiences, not commonly associated with 'traditional' medical students, and this can leave them feeling an imposter in the medical school. Understanding the positive impact of diversity is therefore key for students in the development of their professional identity. When working with students on their own identity and promoting inclusivity, it is important to ensure the students' safety and well-being through the creation of safe spaces and ensuring appropriate support using the key considerations in Box 11.1.

Box 11.1   Principles of working safely with student identity and inclusivity

- Agree confidentiality at the start of a session
- Declare the session a 'safe space' where students are reassured that they will not face criticism or harm
- Share something of yourself with the students to show your trust and gain their trust
- Openly enquire about and value each student's identities and experiences
- Help students to relate their personal identity to their professional identity

- Provide support throughout all sessions, as exploring these areas can bring up powerful feelings for participants
- Build in time for reflection and feedback at the end of the session
- Ensure the session is long enough to avoid rushing any student and allow time for students to debrief afterwards if they need to
- Signpost further student support available to them
- Allocate one facilitator for each small group, and another person to be available if someone becomes distressed
- Provide the opportunity for staff to debrief

The Inclusivity Session is an example of how these principles can be applied, providing an ideal opportunity for students to see their own value and the value of others, and helping them develop a deeper understanding of what they all bring to the medical school. These sessions can be held at any time during the student life cycle, but delivery at six to seven weeks into the first semester is a time that has proved particularly helpful for cohort cohesion. This session works well with small breakout groups of about ten participants. It is important not to rush this activity, as things will emerge through the process of talking about and listening to our stories, so they are timetabled for three hours. Sometimes the whole time is not needed, but this ensures no participant is rushed and there is plenty of time for discussion. It is also helpful for the staff involved not to timetable anything for an hour afterwards as often students want to debrief.

The inclusivity session

We habitually interact with people from our own frame of reference, based on our values and biases. At times, this can make it quite difficult to understand others if we are not familiar with their frame of reference. Exploring our different cultural identities in this session will help create a greater under-standing of each other and our values and support us to work together more effectively.

The learning outcomes of this session are to

- Increase self-awareness of the impact of individual cultural identity on per-sonal bias.
- Appreciate the diversity of the cultural identity of others.
- Develop insight into the influence that cultural identity has on cultivating professional identity.

The resources required are A3 paper, coloured pens, facilitators, and time.

Session stages

The task should be undertaken in small, facilitated groups, ideally eight to ten participants. If working with a larger group of students, the introduction and conclusion can be given to the group as a whole.

1 *Introduction.* Explain the purpose and timeframe of this exercise (as outlined above) and let the participants know what is going to happen and what is expected of them (see below). Emphasise that there is no expectation for them to share anything they are not comfortable with sharing. The confidentiality of the session should be addressed before beginning the exercise and participants need to agree that material shared and discussed in the smaller groups should not be repeated or revealed outside of that group.

2 *Drawing the pictures.* Place the students into groups and ask them to individually draw pictures or diagrams that represent or tell the story of their cultural identity. For example, this can include representations of people, flags/geographical references, religion, education, hobbies, pets, depictions of events, attitudes, or attributes. The facilitator also draws aspects of their identity at the same time. This should take around 10–15 minutes.

   It is helpful to state at the beginning that there is no need to have any drawing skills for this activity, but the use of words in the diagrams is discouraged! Drawing together is a great levelling activity so everyone can participate at the beginning and then share a starting point to the exercise. Some participants focus on drawing educational timelines, as this may feel a safe thing to do, however it is good to encourage participants to think more broadly than just their schooling, if they are comfortable to do so. An example drawing is shown in Figure 11.1.

3 *Sharing the pictures.* In their groups, participants take it in turns to hold up their picture and describe the aspects of their identity they have drawn, explaining what is important to them and why. When they have finished describing, the facilitator encourages the group to ask questions or explore aspects of the participant's identity that were presented.

   It is helpful for the facilitator to share the aspects of their identity they have drawn first; this helps builds trust and create the safe space, encouraging others to feel safe sharing.

4 *Reflection and feedback.* You can develop participants' learning from this exercise by asking them to either reflect individually or feed back to the group on the following:

- What have been the main influences on my cultural identity so far?
- Identify one advantage and one challenge that your cultural identity may give you in developing your identity as a doctor.

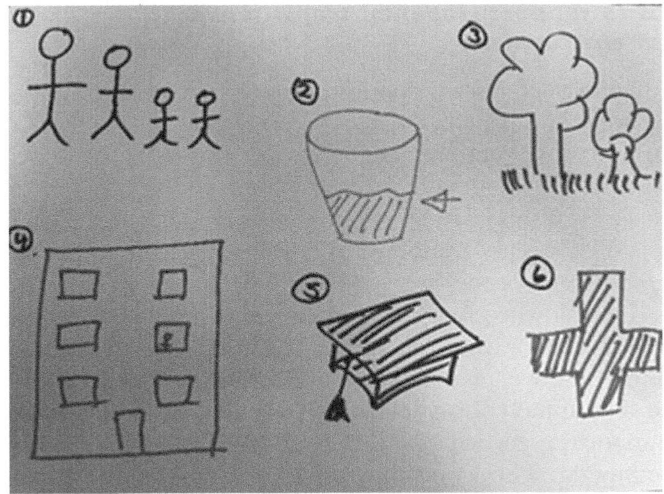

Figure 11.1 An example of a drawing representing aspects of an individual's identity

1 – The family, 2 – 'The glass is half full', representing optimism, 3 – A love of nature and being outdoors, 4 – The individual in a flat, signifying life before university, 5 – A mortar board, representing academic achievements, 6 – A red cross signifying caring responsibilities

5 *Concluding the session*. Either in the small groups or all together, to close the session, you can give participants the opportunity to share any feelings and reflect on taking part in this exercise. You can explain that this kind of activity can bring up strong feelings and encourage participants to stay behind to debrief afterwards if they need to or access external support.

Session support

This session can be triggering for participants, however sensitively it is delivered, so it is important to have support available during and after the session and to signpost students to the support services available to them at the end. It is helpful to have someone who is not involved in facilitating a group to be available to support any student who becomes distressed during the session. Staff may also want to debrief together after the session. Despite all the time this takes and support requirements, it is a hugely fulfilling and rewarding session.

Workshops to support students' transition to the clinical environment

There is little published research on interventions supporting WP medical students during their time at medical school (Cleland et al., 2015). However, examples of institutional interventions designed to increase WP students' self-reported confidence, sense of belonging in medical school, and ability to better manage challenges have been shown to be effective (Kosobuski et al., 2017; Hausmann et al., 2007). WP students' transition to full-time placements can be especially challenging and many of the concerns regarding their legitimacy as a medical student can reappear when faced with entering the clinical environment.

We designed six workshops to help integration into the clinical environment, building on the experiences from the early years of the medical degree programme. This intervention deliberately avoided academic support and focused on supporting participants' self-confidence, professional identity, and sense of belonging. The workshops series was developed to address these needs in the context of the challenges often faced by WP students and were theoretically informed by the principles of self-efficacy, learning through mastery (role-play), vicarious experience (hearing the experiences of graduates), social persuasion (positive support from peers), and emotional and physiological states (developing positive coping strategies) (Bandura, 1994). The six workshops with their respective learning outcomes are outlined in Box 11.2.

These workshops employed the same principles of working with identity and inclusivity as described in the previous section. Each session started by stating the aims of the workshop series, delivering a safety pledge and an outline for that session. Each session was co-facilitated by WP graduates, providing valuable relatable role models. The sessions were optional, held in the evenings and hot food was provided to create a more social atmosphere. Each of the six sessions had two key elements, the first delivered information or theory through practical application, such as role-play or practice conversations. The second element focused on discussion around the relevant topics followed by sharing of experiences, facilitated by the graduates.

The aim of these workshops was to support the transition from a mainly academic environment (university-based) to a predominantly clinical environment (placement-based, e.g., hospital) by enhancing self-efficacy and increasing participants' sense of belonging in the medical school.

The workshops were facilitated by the programme lead of the gateway to medicine programme, (BM6), other key members of the faculty, and graduates of the BM6 programme. Each workshop lasted two hours. The first half of the workshops involved the delivery of, and engagement with, relevant materials and theory around the topic areas. The second half of the workshops was more interactive: clinicians and BM6 graduates facilitated small group discussions and shared their own medical education and professional experiences. Using small groups and encouraging students to share their experiences were essential features of the workshops, which aimed to increase participants' social comfort and sense of belonging to the medical school.

Discuss our challenging experiences and helpful approaches.

Box 11.2 The titles and learning outcomes of the six workshop sessions

1 Inclusivity and cultural identity

   - Discuss unconscious bias.
   - Reflect on our identity and consider different perceptions of identity.
   - Share personal experiences of inclusivity, equality, and diversity.
   - Explore our cultural identity and the value of diversity in medicine.

2 Communication skills and having difficult conversations

   - Explore methods of communication including:

     - non-violent communication,
     - perceptual positioning,
     - transactional analysis.

   - Relate methods of communication to personal experiences.
   - Share experiences of difficult conversations.

3 Coping with stress

   - Discuss how to cope best with stress by exploring:
   - Sources of stress.
   - How can stress impact on us and how we react?
   - Coping strategies and how to manage challenging circumstances.
   - Resilience and self-compassion.
   - Share experiences of dealing with stressful circumstances.

4 Managing difficult personal circumstances

   - Discuss managing difficult personal circumstances through exploring:

     a. Our competing interests
     b. What makes them so difficult to manage?
     c. Strategies that may help you with challenging circumstances.

   - Sharing experiences of coping with difficult personal circumstances

5 Preparing for the clinical environment

   - Build on the skills and strategies gained from the previous workshops.
   - Discuss the expectations and concerns regarding learning and working in the clinical environment.
   - Explore expectations of clinicians with regard to students within the clinical environment.

- Share reflections on undergraduate clinical experiences.

6. Building confidence and professional identity

- Build on the skills and strategies gained from the previous workshops.
- Continue to explore the clinical experience.
- What constitutes professional identity? Discussion.
- Explore potential conflicts between professional identity and personal identity.

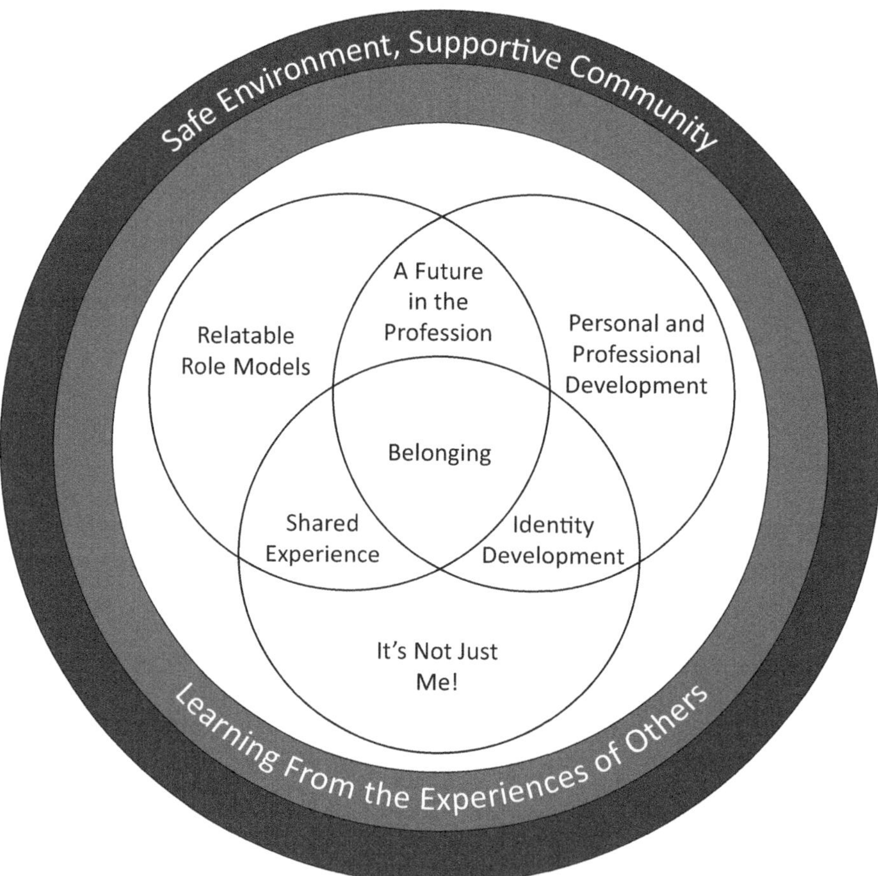

Figure 11.2 The importance of creating a safe and supportive environment to enable the development of a sense of belonging through a series of interacting factors. The relatable role models were especially well-received by the students

A six-month evaluation of the workshops reported (Mozley et al., 2020) that they did support an increased sense of self-efficacy and belonging in participants (see Figure 11.2). A key finding from the evaluation was the importance of the safe environment they were delivered in and how that facilitated the learning and personal development within the workshops. A sense of personal and professional development alongside access to relatable role models and realising, through conversation with peers and facilitators, that others share the same thoughts and feelings were also reported.

Supporting students in developing a sense of professionalism and professional identity is crucial for all students, but for students from under-represented backgrounds with less familiarity with professional culture, particular attention must be paid to the manner of this support. The methods outlined in this chapter demonstrate ways in which medical schools can support WP students with their professional development without subscribing to a deficit discourse model in which students are expected to sacrifice their uniqueness to 'fit in'. By engaging with students on a personal level and encouraging them to embrace their cultural background, medical schools can value students' diversity by supporting them with consolidating their personal and professional identities.

References

Anane, M., and Curtis, S. (2022). Is earning detrimental to learning? Experiences of medical students from traditional and low socioeconomic backgrounds. *The British Student Doctor Journal*, 6(1), 14–22. doi: 10.18573/bsdj.297

Bandura, A. (1994) *'Self-efficacy'*, *Encyclopedia of Human Behavior*. New York: Academic Press.

Boursicot, K., and Roberts, T. (2009). Widening participation in medical education: Challenging elitism and exclusion. *Higher Education Policy*, 22, 19–36. doi: 10.1057/hep.2008.35

Bunce, L., King, N., Saran, S., and Talib, N. (2019). Experiences of Black and Minority Ethnic (BME) students in higher education: Applying self-determination theory to understand the BME attainment gap. *Studies in Higher Education*, 1–14.

Canning, E. A., LaCosse, J., Kroeper, K. M., and Murphy, M. C. (2020). Feeling like an imposter: The effect of perceived classroom competition on the daily psychological experiences of first-generation college students. *Social Psychological and Personality Science*, 11(5), 647–657. doi: 10.1177/1948550619882032

Caruana, V., Clegg, S., Ploner, J., Stevenson, J., and Wood, R. (2011). *Promoting Students' Resilient Thinking' in Diverse Higher Education Learning Environments*. www.advance-he.ac.uk/knowledge-hub/promoting-students-resilient-thinking-diverse-higher-education-learning-environments (accessed 8 March 2024).

Cleland, J. A., Nicholson, S., Kelly, N., and Moffat, M. (2015, January). Taking context seriously: Explaining widening access policy enactments in UK medical schools. *Medical Education*, 49(1), 25–35. doi: 10.1111/medu.12502. PMID: 25545571.

Cotton, D. R. E., Nash, T., and Kneale, P. (2017). Supporting the retention of non-traditional students in higher education using a resilience framework. *European Educational Research Journal*, 16(1), 62–79.

Curtis, S., Mozley, H., Langford, C., et al. (2021, December 24). Challenging the deficit discourse in medical schools through reverse mentoring–Using discourse analysis to explore staff perceptions of under-represented medical students. *BMJ Open*, 11(12), e054890. doi: 10.1136/bmjopen-2021-054890. PMID: 34952883; PMCID: PMC9066338.

Curtis, S., and Smith, D. (2020). A comparison of undergraduate outcomes for students from gateway courses and standard entry medicine courses. *BMC Medical Education*, 20(4). doi: 10.1186/s12909-019-1918-y

Department for Education. (2019). *Impact of the Student Finance System on Participation, Experience and Outcomes of Disadvantaged Young People*. www.gov.uk/government/publications/the-student-finance-system-impact-on-disadvantaged-young-people (accessed 8 March 2024)

Elliott, C. M., Stransky, O., Negron, R., et al. (2013). Institutional barriers to diversity change work in higher education. *SAGE Open*, 3(2), 2158244013489686.

Friedman, S. (2014). The price of the ticket: Rethinking the experience of social mobility. *Sociology*, 48(2), 352–368.

Frost, H. D., and Regehr, G. (2013, October). "I am a doctor": Negotiating the discourses of standardization and diversity in professional identity construction. *Academic Medicine*, 88(10), 1570–1577. doi: 10.1097/ACM.0b013e3182a34b05. PMID: 23969361.

Garrud, P., and Owen, C. (2018). Widening participation in medicine in the UK. In: M. Shah, and J. McKay (eds.), *Achieving Equity and Quality in Higher Education. Palgrave Studies in Excellence and Equity in Global Education*. Cham: Palgrave Macmillan. https://doi.org/10.1007/978-3-319-78316-1_9

Harrison, N., and Hatt, S. (2012). Expensive and failing? The role of student bursaries in widening participation and fair access in England. *Studies in Higher Education*, 37(6), 695–712.

Hatt, S., Baxter, A., and Harrison, N. (2003). The new widening participation students: Moral imperative or academic risk? *Journal of Access Policy and Practice*, 1(1), 16–31.

Hausmann, L. R. M., Schofield, J. W., and Woods, R. L. (2007). Sense of belonging as a predictor of intentions to persist among African American and white first-year college students. *Research in Higher Education*, 48, 803–839. doi: 10.1007/s11162-007-9052-9

Jetten, J., Iyer, A., Tsivrikos, D., and Young, B. M. (2008). When is individual mobility costly? The role of economic and social identity factors. *European Journal of Social Psychology*, 38(5), 866–879.

Kosobuski, A., Whitney, A., Skildum, A., and Prunuske, A. (2017). Development of an interdisciplinary pre-matriculation program designed to promote medical students' self efficacy. *Medical Education Online*, 22, 1. doi: 10.1080/10872981.2017.1272835

Krstić, C., Krstić, L., Tulloch, L., Agius, S., Warren, A., and Doody, G. (2021). The experience of widening participation students in undergraduate medical education in the UK: A qualitative systematic review. *Medical Teacher*, 43(9), 1044–1053. doi: 10.1080/0142159X.2021.1908976

Mathers, J., and Parry, J. (2009). Why are there so few working-class applicants to medical schools? Learning from the success stories. *Medical Education*, 43, 219–228. doi: 10.1111/j.1365-2923.2008.03274.x

McKay, J., and Devlin, M. (2016). "Low income doesn't mean stupid and destined for failure": Challenging the deficit discourse around students from low SES backgrounds in higher education. *International Journal of Inclusive Education*, 20(4), 347–363. doi: 10.1080/13603116.2015.1079273

Medical Schools Council. (2020). *A Guide for Gaining Relevant Experience during the Pandemic*. www.medschools.ac.uk/media/2717/a-guide-for-gaining-relevant-experience-during-the-pandemic.pdf (accessed 8 March 2024)

Medical Schools Council. (2021). *Active Inclusion, Challenging Exclusion in Medical Schools*. www.medschools.ac.uk/media/2918/active-inclusion-challenging-exclusions-in-medical-education.pdf (accessed 8 March 2024)

Mozley, H., D'Silva, R., and Curtis, S. (2020, November). Enhancing self-efficacy through life skills workshops. *Widening Participation and Lifelong Learning*, 22(3), 64–87(24). doi: 10.5456/WPLL.22.3.64

Nazar, M., Kendall, K., Day, L., and Nazar, H. (2015). Decolonising medical curricula through diversity education: Lessons from students. *Medical Teacher*, 37(4), 385–393. doi: 10.3109/0142159X.2014.947938

Patterson, R., and Price, J. (2017). Widening participation in medicine: What, why and how? [version 1]. *MedEdPublish*, 6, 184. doi: 10.15694/mep.2017.000184

Rakestraw, L. (2017). How to stop feeling like a phony in your library: Recognizing the causes of the imposter syndrome, and how to put a stop to the cycle. *Law Library Journal*, 109(3), 465–477.

Reay, D., Crozier, G., and Clayton, J. (2009). "Strangers in Paradise"? Working-class students in elite universities. *Sociology*, 43(6), 1103–1121.

Thomas, L. (2020). Excellent outcomes for all students: A whole system approach to widening participation and student success in England. *Student Success*, 11(1), 1–11. https://search.informit.org/doi/10.3316/informit.579969882009185

Verbree, A. R., Isik, U., Janssen, J., et al. (2023). Inclusion and diversity within medical education: A focus group study of students' experiences. *BMC Medical Education*, 23, 61. doi: 10.1186/s12909-023-04036-3

Warner, R., Hornsey, M. J., and Jetten, J. (2007). Why minority group members resent impostors. *European Journal of Social Psychology*, 37(1), 1–17.

Woolf, K., Potts, H. W. W., and McManus, I. C. (2011). Ethnicity and academic performance in UK trained doctors and medical students: Systematic review and meta-analysis. *BMJ*, 342.

Chapter 12

Contextual admissions in widening participation

Sally Curtis, Clare Owen, and Eliot L. Rees

What are contextual admissions?

Contextual admissions refers to a method used by educational institutions, typically colleges or universities, to consider applicants' backgrounds and personal circumstances alongside their academic achievements when making admissions decisions. The practice of contextual admissions acknowledges the social, economic, and educational challenges and disadvantages that many applicants may have faced. It places their academic achievement within the context within which it was achieved, recognising that an individual's circumstances may not have enabled them with the opportunity to achieve their full academic potential. There has been an increasing use of contextual admissions in the selection and recruitment of medical students over the last 20 years (Medical Schools Council, 2019, 2023), with a notable rise following the recommendations of the Selecting for Excellence Final Report (Medical Schools Council, 2014). This has reflected the national agenda to widen participation to medicine and ensure that the profession is more representative of the population it serves (Medical Schools Council, 2014).

Institutions seek to better understand the context in which applicants' educational achievements have been attained through the use of specific measures. This enables universities to increase the numbers of students enrolled on their courses from social backgrounds that have traditionally been under-represented, by recognising that one of the drivers for this under-representation has been educational disadvantage. Through contextualising prior academic attainment, universities can redress this disadvantage in a data-driven way.

Within medical education, the lowering of academic grade requirements for applicants from lower socio-economic backgrounds is justified by the results of a study of students at 18 UK medical schools. In this study, Mwandigha et al. (2018) found that 'the predictive value of secondary school grades was generally dependent on the secondary school in which they were obtained' meaning that students who performed well at A-level and who went to schools with a high overall academic attainment ultimately performed less well in medical school assessments than students who performed well at A-level and attended a school with lower levels of academic attainment. This led the authors

DOI: 10.4324/9781003399858-12

to suggest that 'the academic entry criteria should be relaxed for candidates applying from the least well performing secondary schools. In the UK, this would translate into a decrease of approximately one to two A-level grades.'

The groups that are under-represented in medical education vary globally depending on the specific context and history of different countries. In Australia, New Zealand, and Canada, an emphasis is put on increasing the participation of students who come from Indigenous and remote and rural communities (Puddey et al., 2017; Curtis et al., 2017; Young et al., 2012). In many European countries, the emphasis is on students who come from migrant communities. In the UK, the focus of widening participation is predominantly on students from lower socio-economic backgrounds and therefore this chapter will focus on this particular aspect of disadvantage. Henceforth, we will refer to them as widening participation (WP) applicants.

How are contextual admissions used?

Most UK medical schools use some form of contextual admissions. However, the benefit it confers on the applicant will vary between institutions. There are three common approaches:

- *Reduced threshold for interview.* This can be through guaranteed interviews or reduced thresholds on aptitude tests or prior academic attainment. This enables WP applicants to demonstrate they have the appropriate interpersonal skills and behaviours for a career in medicine. It should be noted that in many cases the student will still need to subsequently achieve the required academic attainment for the course.
- *Eligibility for a Gateway programme.* Gateway programmes are designed for students from WP backgrounds and aim to support transition and integration to medical school and Higher Education through an additional year of education prior to the commencement of the standard five-year programme. The entry requirements for these courses are generally lower than those of a standard entry medicine programme. For example, applicants may need to achieve BBB at A-level rather than AAA. Contextual measures are used to identify eligibility for the gateway course for WP applicants.
- *Reduced entry requirements.* Many schools use contextual admissions to reduce the levels of prior academic attainment required to access a standard medical degree programme. Eligible WP applicants will be given a differentiated offer that will require lower attainment than those from higher socio-economic groups.

Which contextual indicators are available?

In order to employ contextual admissions, institutions need to first decide who is eligible. This necessitates the use of contextual measures, data-driven indicators of disadvantage, that aim to identify individuals from lower socio-economic backgrounds. In the UK, there are a range of different indicators that can be used that measure different aspects of disadvantage. These can be classified into three main levels of measures:

- *Individual- and household-level measures.* These include whether the applicant is the first in their family to enter higher education, whether the applicant's family was eligible for means-tested state benefits including free school meals, or whether the applicant is a caregiver or has spent time in state care.
- *School-level measures.* These include whether the applicant attended a state, private, or selective school or the average academic attainment of the school the applicant attended. These measures look at the quality of education an applicant received.
- *Area-level measures.* These include measures that look at the number of young people accessing higher education in a specific area, for example, TUNDRA (Tracking UNdeRrepresentation by Area) and POLAR (Participation of Local Areas) (Office for Students, 2021), and the levels of deprivation within the area that the applicant comes from, for example, IMD (Index of Multiple Deprivation). (Medical Schools Council, 2018b)

How do medical schools access contextual indicators?

There are a number of ways that schools can access these indicators and the ease of access, and therefore the resources needed to obtain them, will vary depending on the measure. In the UK, applicants to medical school use a national service called UCAS (Universities and Colleges Admissions Service) to apply. As part of their application, they provide a range of personal data, some of these data are available to medical schools when considering their application and some are not. Through UCAS, medical schools receive self-reported data on whether the applicant is the first in their family to attend higher education, the TUNDRA or POLAR rating of the area they come from, and whether the applicant has been in care.

For other measures, medical schools often must contact the student directly to find out whether they meet the indicator, an example is whether the applicant's family have ever been eligible for means-tested state benefits. These data also need to be validated which requires additional resource.

Schools may also use their own resources to take information obtained through UCAS or their own data collection to find out additional information such as the average performance of the school the applicant attended.

Are all measures equally robust?

Each measure has its own strengths and weaknesses, and no one measure can accurately identify if a student comes from a lower socio-economic background.

Some measures, such as TUNDRA or POLAR, are easily available but can produce false positive results when used in isolation as not all areas of measurement contain people from only one socio-economic background (Boliver et al., 2021). Other measures, such as first in family to attend higher education, are self-reported and therefore should be treated with caution. The most accurate measures are those that relate to the individual and have been externally validated but these are often the most resource-intensive to collect. One proxy measure that fulfils these requirements is eligibility for the UCAT (University Clinical Aptitude Test) bursary. UK applicants who can evidence that they (or their parent/guardian) have been in receipt of means-tested benefits are eligible to apply for a UCAT bursary. Their evidence is verified by UCAT and this information is made available to medical schools along with their UCAT scores. Given this context, it is important that medical schools combine measures to contextualise individuals in the most effective and accurate way.

How can schools combine measures?

Curtis et al. (2014) demonstrated the effectiveness of using a minimum of two contextual factors in recruiting WP students. Data from an established gateway programme with a bespoke admissions process showed majority of WP students recruited using contextual admissions were in the lowest household income category. Over 99% of these applicants had fulfilled at least one externally referenced means-tested criterion.

The organisation Supporting Professionalism in Admissions (SPA) recommended that universities should triangulate the measures used in contextual admissions (Bridger et al., 2012), and this was supported by the Medical Schools Council in its guidance to medical schools; *Indicators of good practice in the use of contextual admission* (Medical Schools Council, 2018b).

A combination of two or three factors from each level of measures (individual, education/school, and geographical, see Figure 12.1) was recommended as being the most effective way of using contextual measures. Boliver et al. (2021) suggest 'the use of administratively verified individual-level metrics to identify contextually disadvantaged learners, most notably receipt of free school meals and low household income'.

Practice – how are contextual admissions operationalised?

When considering contextual admissions in practice, there are two main challenges. Firstly, determining who will have had social, financial, and educational disadvantage and require their application to be considered within this context. Operationally, this means who would be eligible for contextual admissions. Secondly, how to act on this information and alter the admissions process for those eligible applicants (i.e., for those eligible for contextualised admissions, what is the outcome?).

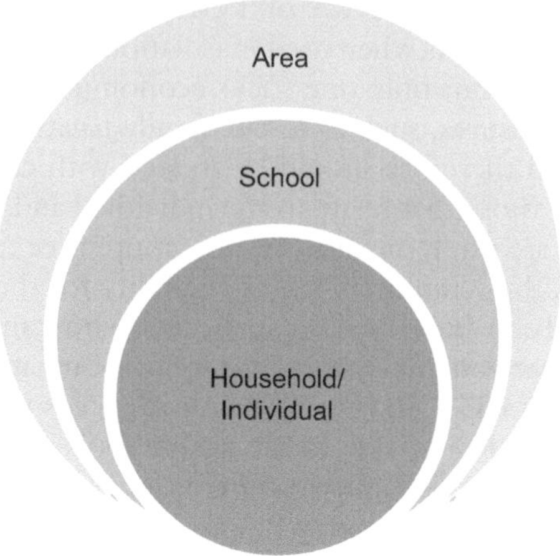

Figure 12.1 Triangulation of contextual measures using different levels of data is more likely to accurately reflect applicants' backgrounds. Some measures clearly reflect individual circumstances and others relate to the household but there can be overlap between them

In 2020, a review of the contextual criteria used in all UK medical schools was conducted based on information publicly available on their websites (Rees et al., 2020). Data was captured using the NCapture function of NVivo and then coded using the categories described by Boliver et al. (2017) as an initial coding framework.

Table 12.1 illustrates the combinations of contextual criteria used by different UK medical schools to determine eligibility for contextual admission for their five-year standard entry medical programmes. At the time of data collection, there were 39 programmes. The majority (29/39, 74%) of these programmes had some form of contextual criteria detailed on their website. Most of these (20/29) had followed the Medical Schools Council guidance in having used at least one criterion in each of the individual, area, and school levels. Half of the programmes used participation in their widening participation scheme as a criterion.

Looking at the individual criteria used by different medical schools within each level, more variability starts to emerge. Table 12.2 illustrates the individual-level criteria used by each standard entry five-year programme. It is clear that different medical schools are using different criteria. Some criteria are used by many medical schools (e.g., has spent time in care) while others are seldom used (e.g., traveller background).

Within individual criteria, the way in which they are defined varies by different medical schools. Ten medical schools used 'low household income' as a criterion. How this was defined varies widely between different medical schools. Examples of the range include

- 'From a household with a gross annual income of £25.00 or below.'
- 'Your combined household income is under £35.00 per year, excluding government benefits.'

Table 12.1 Levels of contextual criteria used by different UK medical schools for standard entry five-year programmes. Each row represents a different medical school. Shaded boxes indicate that at least one criterion at that level is used by the medical school to confer eligibility for contextual admissions

Individual level	Area level	School level	WP Scheme
X	X	X	
X	X	X	
X	X	X	
		X	X
X	X	X	
X	X	X	X
	X	X	
X	X		
X	X		
X	X	X	
X	X	X	X
X	X	X	X
X	X	X	X
X	X		X
X	X	X	
X	X	X	X
X		X	
X	X	X	X
X	X	X	X
X	X	X	
X	X	X	X
X	X	X	X
X	X	X	X
X	X	X	X
		X	
X	X		X
X	X	X	X
		X	
	X	X	

Use of contextual criteria

- 'Your annual household income is below £42,875.'
- 'Have a household income that is below the national average (£42,875 or less before tax).'
- 'Your family income is below £46,350 per year.'

As you can see, for some medical schools, the threshold for low household annual income is almost half that of others. For many medical school

Table 12.2 Individual-level criteria used by different UK medical schools for standard entry five-year programmes. Each row represents a different medical school. Shaded boxes indicate that criterion is used by the medical school to confer eligibility for contextual admissions

FREE SCHOOL MEALS	Low household income	No parental higher education	Parents non-professional job	Has spent time in care	Long-term carers	Traveller background	Refugees, asylum seekers	Disability	Educational disruption	Estraged
				x	x					
x	x	x		x	x			x		x
x	x	x		x						
x	x			x						
				x						
x				x						
				x						
		x		x	x				x	
				x	x		x			
				x						
				x						
				x						
	x	x		x						
x	x			x	x					
				x						
x	x	x		x	x		x			
x	x	x		x					x	
x	x	x		x	x	x	x	x		x
				x						
x	x	x	x	x	x			x	x	x
				x			x			
				x			x			
x	x									
				x	x					x
				x	x					

applicants from lower socio-economic backgrounds, proximity to home is the most important factor when deciding which medical schools to apply to (Rees et al., 2022; Harrison et al., 2022). Variation in the ways that medical schools operationalise contextual admissions, therefore, can lead regional variation in the extent to which applicants need to be disadvantaged in order to be eligible for contextual admissions at their most proximal medical school.

The ways in which the criteria are used also vary. There are several different ways they can be used:

- A single criterion that confers automatic eligibility for contextual admissions (this is often seen for those who have been in state care due to the profound educational disadvantage associated).
- Essential criteria must be met plus a minimum number of other criteria (e.g., must attend state-funded schools plus meet at least two other criteria from a list of eight).
- Minimum number of criteria met (e.g., must meet at least three criteria from a list of twelve, with no essential criteria).
- Criteria in different levels met (e.g., must meet at least one individual-level, one school-level, and one area-level criterion from a specified list).

As demonstrated, there is significant variability in the criteria different medical schools use, how they define these, how they make decisions based on these criteria, and the implications for applicants who meet these criteria. This variability has both advantages and disadvantages. On the one hand, variation means that medical schools can tailor their contextual admission systems to their local context and the forms of disadvantage most pertinent to their settings. It also results in the recruitment of applicants from a wider range of disadvantaged backgrounds, therefore increasing both access and opportunity. On the other hand, variability can cause confusion. Medical schools have not always been completely transparent in the criteria they use and how they use them (Rees and Woolf, 2020). Even when they are, the details can be overwhelming to potential applicants having to consider 40 different medical schools and the different combinations of different criteria used.

Do contextual admissions work?

The UK has used contextual admissions as part of a strategy to increase the number of students from lower socio-economic backgrounds studying at UK medical schools. Representation has improved over the last decade. It would be fair to attribute some of this increase to the use of contextual admissions, whilst also acknowledging that outreach and other activities to attract more applicants from these groups will have played a part. Although there has been an increase in students from lower socio-economic backgrounds, the numbers are still small (Medical Schools Council, 2017, 2018a, 2019, 2023).

Implications of contextual admissions

Individual implications

Attracting and recruiting students from low socio-economic backgrounds to higher education, and specifically medicine, comes with a responsibility to ensure, wherever possible, they are not exposed to further disadvantage during their time at university and in preparation for their future careers. This begs the question, what happens to the understanding, acknowledgement, and adjustments made for an individual's socio-economic and educational background, seen in contextual admissions process once they take up their place at medical school? The familial, social, and financial aspects of a WP student's background continue when they enter medical school and therefore many of the challenges associated with being a WP applicant are relevant, and often more so, to the WP student. Many students from WP backgrounds navigate their way through medical school and university life alongside additional responsibilities for themselves and their families. In addition, it is not uncommon that such challenges can be exacerbated by being at university, it can become more difficult to manage their responsibilities to family members when away from the family home as well as the additional financial requirements and social impact of transitioning to an unfamiliar environment.

Students coming from families with experience of higher education are frequently well supported through, or even shielded from, new and ongoing problems that arise, but WP students are often required to provide support for their families in times of challenge and financial hardship. This was especially notable during the Covid-19 pandemic, with many of our WP students' families being seriously impacted. Students were often expected to take on additional responsibilities such as homeschooling and caring or undertaking increased paid employment to financially support their family. As illustrated by the previous example, WP students' disadvantage is often compounded by intersecting identities, ethnic diversity is higher and parental experience of higher education is lower compared to traditional medical students (Curtis and Smith, 2020). Such considerations can also result in many WP students providing social support for family members on a regular basis, for example helping with translating, dealing with authorities, and administrative tasks or healthcare. Many students travel home at weekends to carry out their roles, which places an additional burden on them, financially due to travel costs and/or educationally due to reduced time available for study. Some WP students find themselves prioritising paid employment over their education to survive and in some cases to support their families (Anane and Curtis, 2022). Such challenges are normally present for most, if not all, of their educational experience. It is worth noting that WP students on six-year courses accrue an additional year's debt for tuition fees and living expenses and are in receipt of the NHS bursary for an additional year, compared to their standard entry counterparts.

For many years, there has been an acknowledgement of acute challenges experienced around the time of exams for all students through processes such as extenuating circumstances or special considerations, which are frequently applied for to mitigate against the impact on exam performance. However, many of the challenges associated with being from a WP background do not suddenly appear around the times of exams, and the student will have usually experienced these throughout their time at school and college. These long-term challenges are likely to have a far more disadvantageous impact on a student's ability to pass exams and progress. Unlike extenuating circumstances, seen for acute challenges, there is often no clear mechanism to mitigate for the long-term challenges faced and the impact on assessments and ultimately, progression. The expectation by many institutions is for students to manage their own long-term challenges. It is important to recognise, however, that not all WP students have ongoing disadvantage and that non-WP students can also experience the same challenges as WP students and can get overlooked and be unsupported.

Institutional implications

For many years, most medical students were white, affluent, and well-educated, reflected by the disproportionate numbers of students from selective and private schools entering medical school (Medical Schools Council, 2014). Consequently, this has created expectations of the medical schools around the previous educational and social experience of medical students, as well as the levels of family support in preparing for university and while studying.

The changing demographic of medical students seen largely through widening participation initiatives over the last 20 years places a responsibility on universities and the medical profession. This responsibility is to ensure that WP students are not additionally disadvantaged by studying medicine in an environment that does not acknowledge or accommodate the circumstances of their background and how that affects their experience as a medical student.

The first six-year widening participation, or Gateway, programmes were launched in the early 2000s and many viewed these as wonderful opportunities that universities were providing for WP students. Once students had enrolled on the programmes, it was commonly assumed they should be able to make the most of this opportunity, to adapt, cope, and progress. It was viewed as a golden opportunity for the students and seen as their responsibility to adapt and assimilate into the university's expectations, and consequent policy and processes, of a 'typical' medical student.

This revealed a tension between the need to diversify the medical profession, ensuring it is more representative of the population, and expecting WP students to assimilate into the role of a 'typical medical student' reducing the impact of their uniqueness and resulting diversity (Razack et al., 2015).

It has become apparent that this short-sighted institutional approach to widening participation can perpetuate disadvantage in several ways. It does not acknowledge the context of the student's background post-admissions. Therefore, the student's performance or experience was not situated in their context but in the context of the expectations of the university, based on affluent, well-educated, and well-supported students. This results in unrealistic expectations and a failure to recognise how the challenges that WP students face impact on their ability to study and focus. Concerns regarding attendance, performance, progression, or retention are frequently attributed to the student's perceived deficits and lack of ability, rather than the competing interests on their time and university's lack of understanding or accommodation of these factors (Curtis et al., 2021). These are all possible contributory factors to the attainment/awarding gap identified in students on gateway programmes compared to their standard entry student counterparts (Curtis and Smith, 2020). Research by Brown et al. (2023) highlights that the attainment/awarding gap is prevalent in medical schools across the UK for students from ethnic minoritised backgrounds. Given the high levels of ethnic diversity in the WP population, this is a widespread problem for students from a variety of under-represented and minoritised backgrounds.

This deficit discourse implies that some students are not as 'good' as others and the impact of being othered, marginalised, unable to speak up, and be themselves. Consequently, this can reduce self-esteem, confidence, and self-belief (Thomas, 2002). It is crucial therefore that universities understand this and stop seeing these students as 'problem students' but rather understanding they are students who are studying alongside additional responsibilities or challenges. It should not be expected that WP students assimilate into an environment that is both unrealistic and unsuitable for them. This is likely to prevent them from bringing and sharing their rich capital and unique experiences with students and staff, helping all understand the diversity of our students, staff, and patients (Beagan, 2005).

It is important to acknowledge that medical schools cannot contextualise assessment outcomes or competency standards for WP students, as seen with the A-level grades on entry. All students, WP or otherwise, must meet the learning outcomes of the medical school and of the outcomes for graduates from the General Medical Council. Medicine is not a classified degree; the aim is to produce competent graduates. However, academic excellence is still coveted by medical schools, being recognised, and rewarded often more so than other attributes of success despite it not being directly related to being a good doctor. This perpetuates and fuels the student deficit discourse for those who have less opportunity to study and prepare for assessments, such as WP students. It is unreasonable to expect WP students to thrive in higher education in the same way as their more advantaged peers, to perform as well and to be able to engage in the same way as students who do not have additional responsibilities and competing interests on their time and focus. The good news is that there are signs the competitive nature of medicine is declining, as seen with the recent move away from academic ranking for UK foundation programme allocation to a preferential allocation system with pre-allocation for WP graduates (Foundation Programme, 2024).

With medical schools inviting and welcoming students from WP backgrounds, as evidenced by the increase in gateway programmes and alternative contextual admissions routes, it is imperative they provide appropriate and sufficient support. As a minimum, they should be acknowledging and understanding the impact of their students' background on their experience at medical school and working to accommodate that within their structures and processes. Supporting WP students appropriately during their undergraduate medical studies will maximise opportunities for them to feel a sense of belonging and to reach their potential.

References

Anane, M., and Curtis, S. (2022, December). Is earning detrimental to learning? Experiences of medical students from traditional and low socioeconomic backgrounds. *British Student Doctor Journal*, 6(1), 14–22. doi: 10.18573/bsdj.297

Beagan, B. L. (2005, August). Everyday classism in medical school: Experiencing marginality and resistance. *Medical Education*, 39(8), 777–784. doi: 10.1111/j.1365-2929.2005.02225.x. PMID: 16048620.

Boliver, V., Crawford, C., Powell, M., and Craige, W. (2017). *Admissions in Context: The Use of Contextual Information by Leading Universities*. London: The Sutton Trust.

Boliver, V., Gorard, S., and Siddiqui, N. (2021). Using contextual data to widen access to higher education. *Perspectives: Policy and Practice in Higher Education*, 25(1), 7–13. doi: 10.1080/13603108.2019.1678076

Bridger, K., Shaw, J., and Moore, J. (2012). Fair admissions to higher education: Research to describe the use of contextual data in admissions at a sample of universities and colleges in the UK. *Supporting Professionalism in Admissions*.

Brown, C., Goss, C., and Sam, A. H. (2023). Is the awarding gap at UK medical schools influenced by ethnicity and medical school attended? A retrospective cohort study. *BMJ Open*, 13, e075945. doi: 10.1136/bmjopen-2023-075945

Curtis, E., Wikaire, E., et al. (2017). Examining the predictors of academic outcomes for indigenous Māori, Pacific and rural students admitted into medicine via two equity pathways: A retrospective observational study at the University of Auckland, Aotearoa New Zealand. *BMJ Open*, 7, e017276. doi: 10.1136/bmjopen-2017-017276

Curtis, S., Blundell, C., Platz, C., and Turner, L. (2014). Successfully widening access to medicine: Part 1: Recruitment and admissions. *Journal of the Royal Society of Medicine*, 107(1), 341–346.

Curtis, S., Mozley, H., Langford, C., et al. (2021). Challenging the deficit discourse in medical schools through reverse mentoring–Using discourse analysis to explore staff perceptions of under-represented medical students. *BMJ Open*, 11, e054890. doi: 10.1136/bmjopen-2021-054890

Curtis, S., and Smith, D. (2020). A comparison of undergraduate outcomes for students from gateway courses and standard entry medicine courses. *BMC Medical Education* 20(4). doi: 10.1186/s12909-019-1918-y

Foundation Programme. (UKFP). https://foundationprogramme.nhs.uk/programmes/2-year-foundation-programme/ukfp/ (accessed 20 January 2024)

Harrison, D., McManus, I. C., Rees, E. L., and Woolf, K. (2022). Institutional choice among medical applicants: A profile paper for The United Kingdom Medical Applicant Cohort Study (UKMACS) prospective longitudinal cohort study. *BMJ Open*, 12(9), e060135.

Medical Schools Council. (2014). *Selecting for Excellence Final Report*. www.medschools.ac.uk/our-work/selection/selecting-for-excellence (accessed 20 January 2024)

Medical Schools Council. (2017). *Selection Alliance Annual Report*. www.medschools.ac.uk/our-work/publications (accessed 20 January 2024)

Medical Schools Council. (2018a). *Indicators of Good Practice in the Use of Contextual Admission*. London: Medical Schools Council.

Medical Schools Council. (2018b). *Selection Alliance Annual Report*. www.medschools.ac.uk/our-work/publications (accessed 20 January 2024)

Medical Schools Council. (2019). *Selection Alliance Annual Report*. www.medschools.ac.uk/our-work/publications (accessed 20 January 2024)

Medical Schools Council. (2023). *Selection Alliance Annual Report*. www.medschools.ac.uk/our-work/publications (accessed 20 January 2024)

Mwandigha, L. M., Tiffin, P. A., Paton, L. W., et al. (2018). What is the effect of secondary (high) schooling on subsequent medical school performance? A national, UK-based, cohort study. *BMJ Open*, 8, e020291. doi: 10.1136/bmjopen-2017-020291

Office for Students. (2021). *Young Participation by Area*. www.officeforstudents.org.uk/data-and-analysis/young-participation-by-area/ (accessed 29 January 2024)

Puddey, I., Playford, D., and Mercer, A. (2017). Impact of medical student origins on the likelihood of ultimately practicing in areas of low vs high socio-economic status. *BMC Medical Education*, 17(1). doi: 10.1186/s12909-016-0842-7

Razack, S., Hodges, B., Steinert, Y., and Maguire, M. (2015, January). Seeking inclusion in an exclusive process: Discourses of medical school student selection. *Medical Education*, 49(1), 36–47. doi: 10.1111/medu.12547. PMID: 25545572.

Rees, E. L., Alexander, K., Mattick, K., and Woolf, K. (2020). Selection in context: The use of contextual criteria in UK medical school admissions. *Association for Medical Education in Europe (AMEE) AMEE 2020: The Virtual Experience*.

Rees, E. L., Mattick, K., Harrison, D., Rich, A., and Woolf, K. (2022). "I'd have to fight for my life there": A multicentre qualitative interview study of how socio-economic background influences medical school choice. *Medical Education Online*, 27(1), 2118121.

Rees, E. L., and Woolf, K. (2020). Selection in context: The importance of clarity, transparency and evidence in achieving widening participation goals. *Medical Education*, 54(1), 8–10.

Thomas, L. (2002). Student retention in higher education: The role of institutional habitus. *Journal of Education Policy*, 17(4), 423–442. doi: 10.1080/02680930210140257

Young, M. E., Razack, S., et al. (2012). Calling for a broader conceptualization of diversity: Surface and deep diversity in four Canadian medical schools. *Academic Medicine*, 87(11), 1501–1510. doi: 10.1097/ACM.0b013e31826daf74

Understanding the impact of identity, inclusion, and recognition on engagement at a small medical school

Single institute case study

Louise Alldridge

Introduction

A GMC survey of the background of postgraduate doctors (General Medical Council, National Training Survey, 2013) revealed the continued and severe under-representation of the working class in the Medical Profession. In relation to this, two further government reports (Milburn, 2012, 2013) highlighted the need for fair access to medicine, the positive implications of a diverse medical workforce on the nation's health, and recommended using evidence of best practice to open access to under-represented groups.

This study was conducted in the setting of a small Medical School prior to a National drive Widen Participation to diversify the medical workforce through the introduction of new medical schools, gateway years, and, more recently, apprenticeship programmes. These welcome initiatives have resulted in an increased proportion of 'non-traditional' medical students from lower socio-economic, refugees, care leavers, carers, and mature student background. This increase in diversity, whilst extremely welcome, brings the need to ensure our pedagogy remains reactive and inclusive and fit for purpose. Much of the focus of Widening Participation (WP) remains on selection processes; alternative entry requirements linked to markers of disadvantage and the introduction of new schools and gateway years. Despite this recent diversification of the medical student body, the way medical students learn and are assessed has largely remained the same.

Pedagogy refers to the methods and practices of an educator, their teaching style, the feedback given, and the assessments they set and review. Inclusive practices and recognition of 'ability' impact significantly on pedagogical experiences and are important considerations for the diverse cohorts created by WP

In this study Traditional Students refers to Medical Students from traditional backgrounds – that is, upper or middle class and usually privately educated. Non-Traditional students refer to those from groups under-represented in medicine and other elite programmes and are usually from working class, and state educated backgrounds.

DOI: 10.4324/9781003399858-13

in medicine. Exclusion and discomfort in learning spaces and misrecognition of ability influence the chances of success for students from non-traditional backgrounds. 'Habitus' is a key concept and is nurtured in the form of dispositions, or trained capacities that influence ways of 'thinking, feeling, and acting' (Bourdieu, 2006). Symbolism of specific cultural, social, and economic capital can be reinforced or rejected in different pedagogical settings.

This single institution study addresses medical pedagogical practices and provides an evidence base to address cultural and social differences. It focuses on the relationship between student and educator identity, and how these impacts on inclusion/exclusion, and success/failure within a medical school. Pedagogical considerations include the impact of teaching medicine through small interactive groups, the expectations linked to practical, clinical, and professional knowledge and skills and a significant requirement for self-directed learning. Inclusive classrooms and physical spaces (including clinical skills spaces and clinical placements) and pedagogies need to be reactive to the current drive to diversify medical students and the ways in which the identities of clinical and academic educators and students might influence 'academic engagement' and assessment. Summative assessment of Professionalism including communication skills and reflective practice are potentially more sensitive to differences in educator and student identities.

The key questions explored by this study included:

a   How do students and educators engage with pedagogy?
b   Can identity, connected with social inequality, influence pedagogical practice?

This chapter builds on research in WP in medicine, HE generally (Crozier and Reay, 2008; Archer et al., 2002), and other 'elite' programmes such as Art and Design (Burke and McManus, 2009), and investigates experiences of pedagogical practice to identify aspects that support or impede the learning and assessment of medical students from different backgrounds. The data was gathered from students and educators to enable consideration and development of inclusive practices in medical education, and to address any challenges of in/equity and mis/recognition of worth and ability in this profession. Medical Schools will be able to refer to this work to support and develop medical students from the broadest range of social backgrounds through consideration and development of inclusive learning for increasingly diverse learners.

Methodology

Theoretical framework

Critical sociology aims to understand structures of domination that can be constraining. Critical sociology of Higher Education underpins this single institute case study through investigation and understanding of the processes of inclusion and exclusion in medical education. Key concepts include identity and recognition of ability and suitability. Pedagogies are undoubtedly influenced by power relations, the changing contexts in which teaching and learning occur, and the changing identities and relations of teachers and students. Medicine, as an elite profession, has the propensity to foster political, social, and cultural power relations across the varied contexts of the curriculum.

Recognition is central to processes of identity formation. Nancy Fraser (1997) stated that to be misrecognised is 'to be constituted by institutionalised patterns of cultural value in ways that prevent one from participating'. For many years, discourses and policies have created a particular understanding of 'Medicine', and what it means to be a 'Doctor' or a 'medical student'. These perceptions can significantly influence educational policies and practices as evidenced in the elite field of Art and Design (Burke and McManus, 2009), where misrecognition of the WP subject through polarising discourses and beliefs lead to exclusion based on false assumptions that these students lacked aspiration, motivation, and/or potential.

In addition, the meaning of 'potential' is often used to serve the interests of privileged groups in society. For example, research on admissions practices in elite Art and Design courses reveals that 'potential' is shaped by 'masculine, middle-class and White racialised' values, subjectivities, and judgements (Burke and McManus, 2009). Like Art and Design, Medicine is an elite programme of study that leads to an elitist profession. It is also dominated and shaped by masculine middle- and upper-class values. The relationship between social inequalities, identities, processes of selection and exclusion, academic achievement, educational choice, and life chances have been relatively overlooked but are now beginning to be acknowledged in medical education (Bochatay et al., 2021). It is important to understand how social and cultural structures, and practices help to perpetuate pedagogical inequalities, misrecognitions, and exclusions. This study looks at the relationship between student and medical educator experiences, their identities and the social structures and cultural practices that are key in the reproduction of dis/advantage, in/equity, and mis/recognition. These considerations are pivotal for all medical educators in the current diversification of medical students through WP.

Research tools

Semi-structured individual interviews were used to collect data from students and educators. Individual student interviews explored access to Medicine and learning experiences, identities, and perceptions whilst individual interviews with clinical and non-clinical educators explored their teaching experiences and perceptions of students in a variety of settings.

Data analysis

Data was analysed in relation to the study questions, drawing on theoretical perspectives on identity formation, recognition, diversity, inclusion, and HE Pedagogy. Using NVivo, preliminary codes were developed, and inductive thematic analysis was used to analyse the different interview transcripts. Emerging patterns and themes of pedagogical experiences perceived by both the educators and the students were noted, reviewed, and named.

Key findings

How do educators engage with pedagogy?

Engagement of educators in pedagogical spaces was strongly influenced by their own identity and the identity of other educators on the programme.

Identity (inter-educator identity)

> I sometimes feel there is a barrier that I'm not a clinician, particularly with some of the hierarchy, there is this kind of clinical/academic divide.

Educator identities are linked to different social and cultural capital (Habitus) which influences engagement with medical school pedagogies including teaching style and perceptions of student ability. As a consequence, educators felt that a hierarchy within the medical school effected recognition of their own talent and worth by students which led to differential student engagement between the two 'classes' of educators.

> I do think that they (clinical educators and students) feel that I don't have the experience that other people have, or I don't have the background that other people have.

An unexpected thread was the strong identity groups amongst educators themselves, which manifested in educator inclusion/exclusion in the workplace. Many of those interviewed remarked on a hierarchy within the medical school and its effect on mis/recognition of educators' own talent and subsequent progression. This hierarchical structure, associated to educator roles, was compounded by a deficit label of 'Non-Clinical Educator' for lecturers without clinical qualifications but with PhDs and significant expertise in Biomedical, Psychological, and Social sciences. This deficit title sometimes manifested in negative experiences for academic Medical Educators:

> A particular person who is a Clinician clearly had an issue that I was academic not clinical and was quite belittling in some of the things that *they* said.

The clinical/academic divide was also seen to intersect with gender identity. The following quotes are from educators who are female and noticed a gender-based culture that impacted on recognition of worth and also exclusion, including opportunities for career progression.

> I would say there is a gender hierarchy, most senior staff are male, so people in power are male.
>
> There are some really hierarchical, archetypal male chauvinists up at the top end of our organisation who think that there's only one way to do things and it's their way.

The same educator completed the comment with:

> It's not everywhere and it's not all men and it's not all women, there are some very nice people who are inclusive, and do help each other and pull people up rather than pushing them down.

Unsurprisingly, intersection with class was also noted. One educator alluded to a class influence on the clinical/academic divide.

> Maybe a class thing, so it's a kind of (they're) standing on a pedestal.

This perceived stereotyping of educators has implications for teaching and learning as students tend to engage more with clinical tutors. In addition, the lack of gender diversity of role models in their clinical education may impact not only on their learning but how they see themselves as clinicians in the future. Since this data was collected, there has been a significant transformation aided by the appointment of a female Head of School with a Biomedical background who implemented a significant reshuffle of roles.

How did educators perceive the way students engaged with pedagogy?

In the previous section, the 'classification' of educators was inferred to influence enhanced engagement in clinical sessions and placements and lower engagement of students in biomedical, sociological, and psychological sessions. Further complex and widespread influence on student engagement in curricular, extracurricular learning and social spaces was noted by Educators to manifest in exclusion in multiple settings through homophilic groupings.

Student identity (educator perception)

> I think students who have similar backgrounds do tend to gravitate towards each other at the beginning at least.

Identity of the students was a key theme when addressing the educators' perception of student engagement. Several educators referred to the different identities and overt social/cultural/financial grouping of students from early in the programme. Having 'matching' cultural capital aided engagement of students with the teaching and learning style and in learning spaces. One educator noted that the 'louder' students who settle in quickly and engage were from

> White middle-class backgrounds, and very confident.

Expanding on this, most educators noted that student engagement was closely linked to other attributes acquired through 'habitus', which clearly helped them position themselves in medical school.

> I think sometimes coming from a background where you have had privilege and been supported, given that confidence, and not had to fight for anything, helps you get on.

Conversely, when educators spoke about the students from WP backgrounds, they noted the interplay between identity and interaction in pedagogical spaces was very different. Students from working class or non-traditional tended to withdraw, leading to discomfort and disengagement, particularly in small group sessions.

> I think these students definitely feel nervous about speaking up.

Educators remarked on the influence of other cultural capital acquired by students from different backgrounds and how these differences play out in pedagogical spaces.

> I think that sometimes is obvious when you have students who are from perhaps less privileged background, that they don't necessarily know how to talk the talk, they don't talk like doctors, and their language is different.

This quote intimates that there is an expectation from educators, for students to adopt a middle-class way of communicating. Students who have been brought up and educated in a privileged setting are advantaged by skills and dispositions developed through their habitus. Conversely, widening participation students from a different social 'field' have developed a different way of perceiving and reacting which could impact on very different outcomes, particularly for clinical skills and presentation assessments.

'Lost voice'/'loud voice'

> I wonder if voices get lost. If you are a representative of anything, you tend to represent your own voice, your own agenda. Those in the 'background' with really good ideas don't have an opportunity or if they do say it, they don't get represented.

Educators noted that students from WP backgrounds did not have a voice and were held back in certain pedagogical settings and were often overpowered by traditional students who displayed an abundance of self-efficacy acquired through classed social and cultural capital. This also manifested in remarks about non-traditional students being 'shy', 'quiet', and educators noticing a certain amount of 'discomfort'.

> There are students who disengage from certain learning activities and that is difficult, I see people who have opted out really, they're not involved in discussion and maybe because they're shy, or they don't know as much as they feel they should.

WP students remain a minority and in small groups, and their experiences and views may be very contrasting to those of the facilitator and rest of the group. One educator acknowledged:

> Some students come [to small group sessions] just not feeling confident to speak in that kind of setting, certainly not to express a view that is different to the norm, they lack confidence in their own ability and the value of what they want to say.

Conversely, Educators also remarked how the self-efficacy of traditional students helps them to consolidate their position in educational spaces.

> Loud and confident white middle-class students who are told that they are doing really well, I think kind of helps them position themselves.

However, it was also noted that often the most confident did not give as useful contributions.

> The natural speaker-outers, not necessarily the most thoughtful or not necessarily the people with the most important things to say.

Sadly, educators were also aware of bullying behaviour by clinical tutors towards WP students, whose expectations can be classed and related to cultural capital and identity.

> I still hear stories both of students feeling very uncomfortable, for all kinds of reasons during teaching and may well feel they've been picked on or bullied or something and not feeling comfortable or confident to speak.

This *lost voice* theme was also prominent in student interviews, and many quotes alluded to a significant impact on learning for this group of students.

'Being a professional'

At this medical school, 'Professionalism' is developed across the curriculum in a range of settings including small groups, workshops, placements, teamwork, and reflection. The module aims to develop the professional knowledge, skills, and behaviours expected of medical students as well as doctors which are defined by the General Medical Council (GMC). Students must demonstrate and be assessed on professional conduct through 'Professionalism Judgements' across all modules, in a variety of educational settings. In many respects, the expectations of students to be 'professional' are 'classed'.

Giving and responding to critical and constructive feedback are very important skills to acquire in medical school and as a doctor. Educators found that this skill, while relatively easy for those from traditional backgrounds, was a challenge for students from a WP background.

> It is something they find difficult personally. It is cultural they're not familiar with that kind of way of speaking I suppose it's not what they do.

This has inherent issues, in particular who sets the standards of professional behaviour and are these classed/cultural to a certain extent. This was noted by a GP educator, who also alluded to the fluidity of what is 'deemed' professional.

> And I'm also aware that there are cultural differences to professionalism and that is something we haven't really addressed as a school so it's very complex.

As with many medical assessment students whose parents are doctors are seen to have an advantage in medical/clinical exams. Interestingly, the requirement to pass the professionalism module every year appears to have manifested in transformation and conforming of WP students to the expected 'way of being' for Medical Students that both educators and students noted.

Engaging in extracurricular social and learning spaces

An unexpected theme that emerged in educator interviews was overt exclusion/inclusion linked to identity observed in extracurricular spaces. The most striking example was seen in the Medical Society (MedSoc) traditionally run by middle/upper class students. This society offers exclusive and 'classed' activities such as 'Grand Balls' with formal dress codes and overseas summer/skiing trips. One educator remarked on power positioning of students through this society:

> A clique of students run MedSoc, so they have a huge amount of power in the medical school, and it really marginalised students who weren't involved or who didn't want to be friends with that clique.

As well as the 'classed' social aspects of this society, members also ran 'MedSoc Teaches'. These sessions were not ordinarily attended or delivered by students from WP backgrounds, leading to exclusion in pedagogical spaces outside of the formal curriculum. Students from a WP background have set up an alternative 'MedSoc' providing their own teaches and network, creating a distinct division and example of a response to not *fitting in*.

Transforming and conforming

An intriguing and unexpected theme that emerged from educator interviews was the noticeable *identity changes* as students went through medical school. It is possible that this is precipitated partly from the permeation of 'professionalism' across all teaching and learning and the desire to 'fit in' and pass clinical and professional assessments. Several educators commented on a transformation of identity over the years at medical school and particularly from Year 3 where students conformed to the perceived or expected 'identity of a doctor'.

> You can see they start trying to talk like doctors, whereas I think that some of the ones that perhaps have been brought up with it have learned to use the language and are much more comfortable and it doesn't come across as trying to be more than they are.

This educator, from a traditional background, identifies WP students as deficient in the classed eloquence of peers from upper- and middle-class background whose communication skills have been developed in a habitus matched that of the educator.

From Year 3, most of the teaching and learning at this medical school takes place in a separate (more prestigious) building next to the hospital. Educators commented on the transformation of student identity and a conformation to the perceived normalised identity of a doctor.

> Over there they behave like adults, sit nicely, drink their coffee and that kind of thing, on main campus they had their feet on the table and all the rest of it.

Again, it is possible that these students from non-traditional backgrounds noticed how success was linked to a specific identity and made conscious/unconscious efforts to conform.

In summary, educators noted how their own professional identity and gender influenced perceived achievement and progression as well as respect from and engagement of students. Educators noted that students held clinicians in higher esteem, and this resulted in reduced engagement with educators with an academic background. They also noticed that students with *matching/expected 'capital'* of traditional Doctors were perceived as 'good students' and this most likely influenced assessments, particularly of 'professionalism' due to 'expected ways of being' linked to capital. These identities also played out in power positioning in extracurricular settings.

How do students engage with pedagogy?

Similar to the educator perceptions, student engagement was linked to identity, class, and habitus.

Class and habitus (cultural capital/social capital/ economic capital)

> I feel like if I had some advice at the beginning it would have been easier, it was a struggle, I was so lucky.

Prior to contemplation of the impact within an education setting, many students alluded to advantages perceived in traditional students from upper middle class with matching identity and habitus to the classed selection procedures leading to access to Medical School. Interestingly, selection and admission for medical school were not mentioned by educators who may have been unaware that they and the 'assessment' of candidates recast privilege as merit (Taylor et al., 2023). The process was clearly an important and impactful experience for all; however, difference in experiences reveal a process that produced an 'exclusive' cohort. In general, those from non-traditional background showed resilience and determination, whilst those from more privileged backgrounds were aided by *social capital* accrued from their family (who in many cases had connections to clinical careers), wider contacts/networks, and schools.

Students from a WP background 'fell into' the idea of studying medicine, had very few connections (family or through schools) to help them through the process of application and selection, and mostly attributed their success to *'luck'*.

> I was wandering through town and open day was on, I just wandered in, I was like really interested in all the stuff that was going on, yeah, and then I kind of started looking into it a bit more.

Other students from a WP background remarked:

> I didn't have any friends, who were interested, our school hadn't sent anyone to do medicine before, and nobody in my family is a doctor so it was a bit of a sort of, trial and error I guess, just like finding stuff out.

These comments show the struggle faced by working-class students to access medicine and their perception that luck was a key influence and not their ability.

In contrast, quotes from students from more privileged backgrounds show self-efficacy, confidence as well as 'easier' access to information regarding applications and work experience through social capital.

> I decided that I definitely wanted to do medicine, and I did a lot of work experience to cement that, my sister does medicine in London, she's a third year.

For this student, the decision was never in doubt and was helped by appropriate social capital to gain access to work experience as well as access to *'privileged' information and guidance* on how to navigate the application and selection processes. Another student from a traditional background also displayed significant social capital from family members and a sense of *'rite of passage'* from an early age.

> My mum's side of the family are all medical. I was brought up surrounded by the healthcare profession, it always occurred to me that I would end up in the healthcare profession.

Without these connections, students from WP backgrounds displayed evidence of *determination, drive, and 'nouse'* to seek out and make connections and gain experience in a healthcare setting.

> So, the hospital was near my house, so I just basically rang them up and eventually got through to the right person and applied for it like that.

The students from Working-Class backgrounds demonstrated *resilience* and determination to navigate the application process with no help from schools, families, and friends. Many of the WP students had also applied more than once to medical school. In contrast, those from more affluent backgrounds did not refer to accessing medicine as difficult and used close family connections and/or attended supportive schools that often have 'in-house' Medical Societies to help those interested in medicine.

Student identity at medical school

Once in medical school, student identity plays a key part in integration, group formation, and learning. Akin to educators, students also talked about identity formations linked to class and habitus. The inherent confidence of middle, upper class students, referred to as traditional students, in this research, appears to confer a pedagogical advantage. A dominant theme for students was *having influence*, and this was generally linked to the *cultural capital* acquired by traditional students through schools, families, and other connections. This group of students had *'the right' voice* and therefore influence. Certain cultural cues were perceived as meritorious and related to success at medical school.

As with the educators, students also noticed the *'lost voice'*, for those from WP backgrounds, and the influence gained by traditional students.

Having a 'voice' and influence

'Students' from 'traditional background' who are quite confident, get the fact that they can influence things and that they have got a voice, and I think this is a lot to do with their education and their culture, if you've come up through a private education, then you're more likely to understand that you do have a voice. Other cultures and different classes perhaps don't have the same voice.

(WP Student)

This equates with the educator comments about contributions in pedagogical spaces and regarding other positioning, such as Year Reps and 'MedSoc' committee members, and the power it holds. Having a voice in many settings which included Student Staff Liaison committees and Curriculum Theme Groups means this 'group' of students can influence the curriculum to suit their background and perhaps not those from WP backgrounds.

Fitting in: inclusion and exclusion

I was shocked with the amount of people who had gone to private school, that was kind of one of my initial thoughts actually, I'd never met somebody that had gone to a private school before, and like it was a bit of a culture shock.

(WP Student)

The difference in backgrounds and therefore social and cultural capital between traditional students and those from WP background played a role in fitting in at medical school and consequently on their engagement with a somewhat classed pedagogy. Many of the WP students talked about exclusion. The student quoted above, clearly felt like an *outlier* and the reference to 'culture shock' illustrates the powerful impact of being 'different'.

Students noticed that exclusion in physical spaces was also evident. One student from a non-traditional background talked about physical segregation/exclusion in accommodation that was clearly associated with class and financial capital:

Here is a bit of a funny thing there is a more expensive Hall [student accommodation], like thirty quid more a week, so already there was this sort of a divide, choosing one was a sort of financial sort of trait.

This quote also indicates a material divide, linked to *'Financial Capital'* acquired through 'habitus', categorising the 'haves' and 'have nots' from the outset of their journey to become doctors.

An abundance of confidence and subsequent power positioning clearly helped traditional students to *'fit in'* with the culture of Medical School. As noted in educator interviews, this student talked about MedSoc and how it helped them fit in.

> We all got on so well and we all clicked and bonded really early on, and by the end of the first week I already felt so comfortable.

Conversely, when students from widening participation backgrounds were asked if they felt like part of the medical school one of the students categorically felt they did not and still showed signs of not fitting into the 'culture'.

> No, I don't know why though, I don't know really, I feel kind of like no.

Class did however feature in an adverse way for the identity of some students. One widening participation student felt 'labelled'.

> I think I was kind of labelled as a bit more chavvy than most people.

Clinical classrooms and placements were pedagogical spaces that students from widening participation backgrounds found particularly uncomfortable.

> Starting third year you are thrown into the clinical world it is really scary.

In such environments, their identity, linked to 'capital', is mismatched to the behaviour, responses, confidence, and self-efficacy of many clinical educators. Consequently, these students found clinical placements more intimidating, when compared to spaces within the medical school. It was common at this time for students to experience bullying behaviour. A female WP student relayed an unpleasant experience in Year 3 with a male clinician on a ward during a placement.

> The Doctor completely grilled me; he grilled and grilled me. When I didn't know he just kept asking me more and more questions, in front of like everyone, there was a lot of other people around. I was so thrown and upset I couldn't answer anything, my mind went blank and that was just a really horrible experience.

This student did not have the confidence, and self-efficacy, that was expected by the clinician, to deal with this situation. It illustrates how social power, hierarchy, and social identities can lead to bias in medical education and reinforces the presence of discrimination and harassment in medical education. Regrettably, harassment and discrimination were prevalent around this time in clinical settings. Reporting however was a rare event as it was perceived as ineffective, linking again to the *'lost voice'* and prominent power positioning (Broad et al., 2018). This particular experience also revealed a bullying and humiliating educational experience, which can be very damaging to students' mental well-being (Dahlin et al., 2005) and may impact and be more prevalent in interactions with students from WP backgrounds.

Independent learning

> For me it wasn't too different, I think some people struggled with EBL because you were kind of expected to do your own work . . . obviously, I was used to that, I'd already had two years that I'd had to do all my own work to get into medical school, so I found it easy.
>
> (WP Student)

A large part of the philosophy at this and many medical schools is ensuring students are equipped for lifelong learning. The curriculum at this medical school is integrated, and science is learned in a clinical context from Year 1. In the first two years, Enquiry-Based Learning using cases is the central pedagogical pin, this relies on a considerable amount of self-directed learning. Here, prior knowledge is identified and learning issues are negotiated to form the basis of self-directed learning between the sessions. This leads to a deeper and long-lasting grasp of key principles (Mattick et al., 2004).

Students from WP backgrounds had often attended large poor performing schools and were very comfortable with being independent learners compared to traditional students who were used to being told what they needed to know to pass exams. The students from WP backgrounds also have personal experience to draw on which brings a diversity of knowledge and new learning to these sessions.

Small group learning

Some tension was noted in a small group learning setting with students from traditional and WP backgrounds. This student, from a WP background, found discussions in small groups about political and social aspects of health challenging.

> The biggest thing I probably struggle with is discussing sort of health politics and stuff. Political views can be quite varied, there's also quite a lot of more conservative medics, so, there's people with quite varied views to you which was difficult.

However, this student remarked that her 'day-to-day life' has equipped her to confront contrasting opinions with evidence and diplomacy. This also shows the value of a diverse cohort, particularly in a small group setting, and how education can be enriched through the diversity of the group.

Transforming and conforming

As noted by Educators, medical students also noticed the transformation of their own identity to conform with the expected identity of a 'clinician'. This third-year student from a WP background talked openly about her 'transformation'.

> I now view myself as a doctor, it has become very integral to who I am and that is why we take on these traits, behaviours and attitude because it is the kind of person I want to be and want to be viewed as.

Whilst educators remarked on the identity transformation of students, the students themselves noticed more subtle changes. These changes were also noticed by friends and family on returning home.

> People say I am not so like my friends from home now, they would say I am not like other people doing medicine, but now I would say I am not so different [to people doing medicine] anymore.
>
> (4th-year WP medical student)

Conclusion

> WP means at its most fundamental that I might be developing better doctors, and for me what better doctors mean is very personal to me which is about doctors who are more responsive to the needs of their patients, more respectful of their patients, more patient-centred, more ethical, more socially accountable, more understanding of inequalities, you know all that kind of thing, and obviously expert clinicians, but people who can combine all of those things into being a good doctor.
>
> Clinical Educator

Pedagogies in a medical education setting can reflect class and gender bias of educators, students, and the medical profession. Historical expectations of knowledge as well as ways of 'being' impact the ways students and educators engage with each other and pedagogy. For students, the impact of 'difference' began with application to medical school. Once in Medical school, experiences and performance were linked to levels of self-efficacy, confidence to speak up and engage. Identity also influenced power in extracurricular spaces. For educators, this single institute study illustrated the influence of identity linked to 'profession', class, and gender in pedagogical settings.

There is now widespread optimism and positivity as a consequence of a national drive to change the demography of medical students and future doctors. The introduction of a Gateway year at this medical school in 2019 has significantly increased the proportion of WP students. The school is also soon to offer a Medical Apprenticeship Programme. Such progress, here and across the country, highlights the importance of this research. Going forward, we have set up a research group to follow our WP students through their medical degree to gather further information on the pedagogical practices that impede progression for these students as they go through Years 1 to 5.

References

Archer, L., Hutchings, M., and Ross, A. (eds.). (2002). *Higher Education and Social Class: Issues of Exclusion and Inclusion*. London: Routledge Falmer.

Bochatay, N., Bajwa, N. M., Ju, M., Appelbaum, N. P., and van Schaik, S. M. Towards equitable learning environments for medical education: Bias and the intersection of social identities. First published: 26 July 2021 https://doi.org/10.1111/medu.14602

Bourdieu, P. (2006). Cultural reproduction and social reproduction. In: D. B. Grusky, and S. Szelényi (eds.), *Inequality: Classic Readings in Race, Class, and Gender* (pp. 257–271). Boulder, CO: Westview Press.

Broad, J., Matheson, M., Verrall, F., Taylor Anne, K., Zahra, D., Alldridge, L., and Feder, G. (2018). Discrimination, harassment, and non-reporting in UK Medical Education. *Medical Education*, 52(4), 414–426. doi: 10.1111/medu.13529

Burke, P. J., and McManus, J. (2009). *Art for a Few: Exclusion and Misrecognition in Art and Design Higher Education Admissions*. London: National Arts Learning Network.

Crozier, G., and Reay, D. (2008). *The Socio-Cultural and Learning Experiences of Working-Class Students in HE: Full Research Report*. Colchester, Essex: UK Data Archive.

Dahlin, M., Joneborg, N., and Runeson, B. (2005). Stress and depression among medical students: A cross-sectional study. *Medical Education*, 39(6), 594–604.

Fraser, N. (1997). *Justice Interruptus: Critical Reflections on the "Postsocialist" Condition*. London and New York: Routledge.

General Medical Council. (2013). *National Training Survey, Socioeconomic Status Questions 2013*. www.gmc-uk.org/-/media/documents/Report_NTS_Socioeconomic_Status_Questions.pdf_53743451.pdf

Mattick, K., Dennis, J., and Bligh, J. (2004). Approaches to learning and studying in medical students: Validation of a revised inventory and its relation to student characteristic and performance. *Medical Education*, 38(5), 535–534. doi: 10.1111/j.13 65-2929.2004.01836.x

Milburn, A. (2012). Fair access to professional careers. *The Independent Reviewer on Social Mobility and Child Poverty*. https://assets.publishing.service.gov.uk/media/5a78a420e5274a277e68e514/IR_FairAccess_acc2.pdf

Milburn, A. (2013). Social mobility and poverty commission. *State of the Nation: Social Mobility and Child Poverty in Great Britain*.

Taylor, J., Wendland, C. L., Kulasegraram, K., and Hafferty, F. W. (2023). Admitting privileges: A construction ecology perspective on the unintended consequences of medical admissions. *Advances in Health Science Education, Theory and Practice*. (4), 1347–1360. https://pubmed.ncbi.nlm.nih.gov/36856902/

Chapter 14

Widening participation in medicine

Beyond widening access

Mandy Hampshire, Peter Leadbetter, and Monisha Gupta

Introduction

Nationally, there has been a rapid increase in the number of initiatives to widen access to medicine, such as Foundation or Gateway Years and contextual offers for 'standard' Medicine courses. This coincides with government priorities aimed at ensuring that doctors are more representative of the population they serve (HEE, 2014; Medical Schools Council, 2014; Medical Schools Council, 2023). The participation of students from diverse socio-economic, ethnic, and cultural backgrounds is vital for social mobility, economic development, and for a medical workforce that adequately represents the general population (McDuff et al., 2020). Furthermore, in England, Higher Education (HE) institutions are required to develop access and participation plans (OfS, 2019), which support student engagement and participation in learning and teaching, whilst fostering an inclusive academic culture (Mountford-Zimdars et al., 2015; Singh, 2011; Berry and Loke, 2011).

Although it is important to widen access to medicine, a significant challenge is to also enable participation during and after undergraduate medical training for students from widening access backgrounds, as difficulties follow them through medical school and beyond (Curtis and Smith 2020; Krstic et al., 2021). Currently, research and commitment from medical schools and the higher education sector continue to focus on widening access (recruitment) with little emphasis on success whilst studying for a medical degree (Krstic et al., 2021).

We address some of the key issues faced by medical students from widening access backgrounds, of which many are associated with lack of finances. The role of institutional culture and the power of the hidden curriculum are discussed, along with successful initiatives that can support widening access students' participation in the formal medical curriculum. We also highlight the challenges students from widening access backgrounds have when they apply for their first jobs through the UK Foundation Programme. We conclude by exploring further barriers faced following graduation as these students plan for their future career and apply for postgraduate training.

DOI: 10.4324/9781003399858-14

What issues limit participation in medical education for students from widening access backgrounds?

Finance

There are many important issues that hinder full participation in medical student life and success through medical school for students from widening access backgrounds, but the key factor is lack of money. Beyond tuition fees and accommodation/day-to-day living costs, students need a level of financial support to participate in social activities at university and provision for 'hidden' costs of studying. For medical students, there can be additional costs, such as expensive stethoscopes, smart clothes to wear on clinical placement, or the expectation that students will buy their own 'scrubs'/clinical uniform. There can also be costs associated with travel to and from clinical placements, buying food while on placement, and potential costs linked to accommodation. Although students may be reimbursed for travel costs, those who don't have a car, or the privilege of a driving licence, can be forced into relying on public transport, that can make commutes to placements lengthy and unpredictable in comparison to the convenience of driving. Clinical placements can mean longer or irregular hours and placements away from where students 'normally' live, making it more difficult for medical students to have paid employment.

As medicine courses are longer than most university courses, more years are spent living as students prior to receiving paid work as a doctor. In addition, medicine courses, particularly in the clinical years frequently include shorter holidays and minimal non-timetabled time, meaning less opportunity for medical students to be in paid employment. Both factors are a challenge to medical students, particularly those who have limited finances, because they are less likely to have sufficient paid employment to supplement whatever bursaries or loans they may receive.

As medical students in England progress through their course, they will move from Student Finance loans and University bursaries or scholarships onto the NHS bursary, usually for the final one or two years of their course, www.nhsbsa.nhs.uk/nhs-bursary-students. The NHS Bursary pays for university tuition fees and provides a maintenance grant (both non-means-tested and means-tested). Medical students may receive significantly less money when they switch from Student Finance loans to NHS bursary funding and may no longer be eligible to receive university bursaries or scholarships (Lok, 2022; Murray, 2022). Students from widening access backgrounds generally do not have financial support from their family or other sources, so are disproportionately impacted. A recent report has identified that the cost of repaying student loans after graduation and the ability to manage costs while studying put potential students off from applying to healthcare courses at university. A national scheme that would write off some or all tuition fees when graduates start work in the NHS would make young people more likely to study a university-based healthcare course (Dodsworth, 2024).

Many of these students will need to work to earn money, resulting in less time to study. They may also have financial responsibility for others. Such factors contribute considerably to a negative impact on well-being (Anane and Curtis, 2022). This is often invisible and not considered by staff (Foreshew and Al-Jawad, 2022) and consequently impacts learning and progression through failing assessments and poorer health, especially mental health (Anane and Curtis, 2022). Some medical students ask to interrupt their studies, to earn money in order to continue on their medicine course later when it is financially viable. Students often request special consideration when being allocated to clinical placements that are a significant distance from the university/medical school, to reduce costs of travel or to enable them to continue in employment where they are usually based.

> ## Case study – financial support for medical students, University of Nottingham
>
> Until recently, the University of Nottingham offered means-tested support to students from widening participation backgrounds during the early years of their Medicine course. However, these bursaries and scholarships ceased when medical students became eligible for the NHS bursary. Loss of university financial support and reduced maintenance loans could reduce medical students' income by £5,000 per year. Following a campaign initiated by a medical student, Monisha Gupta, supported by Professor Sir Jonathon Van Tam, who was Pro-Vice-Chancellor for the Faculty of Medicine & Health Sciences, the University of Nottingham, altered their 'Core Bursary' eligibility requirements to include all medical students, regardless of their year group or NHS Bursary status. This has resulted in medical students from low-income backgrounds receiving up to an extra £2,000 per year during their final years of study. www.nottingham.ac.uk/studywithus/ugstudy/articles/scholarships-and-bursaries-ug.html

Self-efficacy and belonging

Widening access medical students can lack confidence and a sense of belonging as they study at medical school. This may influence their social life and networking leading to relative isolation that can exacerbate 'imposter syndrome' and hinder professional identity development. There can be an identity conflict where the culture of the medical school is mismatched to working-class background and worldview (Krstic et al., 2021, see Alldridge: Chapter 13). Accounts from these students indicate that they feel marginalised, 'othered', at university, and are likely to experience microaggressions, class stigmatisation by peers, and may feel undervalued and not supported (Foreshew and Al-Jawad, 2022; Messiou, 2012; Munn and Lloyd, 2005; Reay et al., 2010; Meuleman et al., 2015; Soria and Bultman, 2014).

Lack of role models amongst staff or students in more senior years can add to the reduced feelings of belonging (Krstic et al., 2021). Medical students may not identify a need for support and potentially not see themselves as being from a 'Widening Access' background, particularly if they enter their medicine course directly rather than from a Foundation/Gateway Year. If they are aware of being from a lower social background than their peers, they may not want to be seen as different. Relative isolation may result in students having less opportunity to learn from peers via the 'hidden curriculum', that is, informal learning that occurs outside formal teaching, and not having the confidence to seek advice from peers or staff (Krstic et al., 2021).

Success at medical school may also be impacted in other ways for students from widening access backgrounds. For example, they may have personal IT equipment that is outdated, impacting their learning through online resources. Assessments may also rely on students having good IT equipment able to support current versions of software. www.officeforstudents.org.uk/news-blog-and-events/press-and-media/digital-poverty-risks-leaving-students-behind/

The learning skills that medical students arrive with at university can also vary depending on the quality of teaching they have received in secondary school and any additional support they may have had access to at home. www.officeforstudents.org.uk/publications/schools-attainment-and-the-role-of-higher-education/

In summary, staff involved in curricular design, in teaching, or in supporting medical students need to be aware of the financial pressures that may significantly impact the learning and well-being of students from widening access backgrounds, particularly in the later clinical years of their medicine course. Good academic, financial, and personal support should be provided for all medical students so that those from widening access backgrounds do not feel stigmatised and can access support easily. Peer support that is inclusive and fosters a sense of belonging for all medical students is important to help students from widening access backgrounds participate and make the most of opportunities during their undergraduate medical training.

Pedagogy and implications for teaching medicine in higher education

An institutional commitment to widening participation is essential to 'truly' widen participation. This not only includes detailed and committed institutional access and participation plans but also the adoption of a democratic philosophy where educational performance is viewed in terms of structural issues such as social inequality. This moves away from the 'deficit model' where students from widening access backgrounds with lower attainment are viewed as lacking ability or desire. The goal of pedagogy is therefore not only to provide appropriate experiences and extra support but to start from the assumption that Higher Education marginalises widening participation cultures and values (Sheeran et al., 2007).

Consistent with this approach, a 'problem-posing education' is required that asks students to engage in self-directed enquiry to understand the conditions responsible for social inequality (Cavanagh et al., 2019). The aim is to promote a critical consciousness among students where 'rote' memorisation and didactic teaching is predominately replaced by problem-based or case-based learning. This aligns to situated learning and communities of practice where learning is tied to context and occurs through participation and active engagement and considers how learning is influenced by the students' goals, attitudes, values, knowledge, and experience (Mann, 2011). It is a learning curriculum and not a teaching curriculum (Lave and Wenger, 2001). Students work through 'real-world' cases and the teaching and learning are developed to support such cases. This serves a dual purpose of promoting student ownership of medical knowledge and integrates them into the thinking practices (culture) of medicine (Hmelo-Silver and Barrows, 2006). Educators prepare learners for professional roles and develop professionals who are self-aware and continue to be lifelong learners (Mann, 2011).

Furthermore, consistent with inclusivity, the curriculum needs to be accessible, to ensure students see themselves in the curriculum, and equip students with the necessary skills and attributes for medicine (McDuff et al., 2020). Within the design and implementation of the curriculum, consideration needs to be given to the notion that under-represented students in medicine have more negative perceptions of the medical school learning environment than their peers (Nemiroff et al., 2023). Widening participation students are likely to see a disconnect between their identity and the medical school professional identity encouraged via the 'hidden curriculum' (Nemiroff et al., 2023). They often encounter a lack of identifiable role models and can experience negative stereotypical views of patients from socially disadvantaged backgrounds in course content (Krstic et al., 2021). Much of a learner's attitude, behaviour, and identity is shaped by the 'hidden curriculum' in an institution's learning environment (and in associated placement settings). Consideration and careful planning are therefore required to ensure diversity of experiences, role models, and suitability of placement experiences (Yazdani et al., 2020). Awareness of the 'hidden curriculum' and learning environment is required in planning and delivering initiatives that target widening participation students. On a practical level, this involves four recommendations for implementation:

1 Teaching and learning to promote integration (inclusive of individual attitudes, knowledge, and experience).
2 Promoting habits of inquiry and improvement (problem-posing education and real-world cases).
3 Individualising learning, yet standardising assessments, and
4 Supporting the development of student's professional identity via the university culture and the 'hidden curriculum' (Mann, 2011).

> **Case study – the Foundation Year for medicine at Edge Hill University**
>
> Nationally, there are now over 20 Foundation Year or Gateway to Medicine courses. The Foundation Year for Medicine at Edge Hill University is not unique, in that it targets young people from non-traditional backgrounds. Students who successfully pass the Foundation Year are guaranteed direct entry onto Year 1 of Medicine at Edge Hill University, completing a six-year medical degree (as opposed to a standard five-year medical degree). The aim of the Foundation Year at Edge Hill University is to prepare students personally, professionally, and academically for the rigours of medicine. The programme was designed with consideration of Mann's four recommendations (Mann, 2011) and specifically targets young people who meet various widening participation requirements, and do not typically have the desired grades for direct entry to medicine. The programme was also designed with awareness that medicine is still an elite profession with the selection process biasing more privileged groups in society (Grafton-Clarke et al., 2018), that selecting students from disadvantaged backgrounds enriches the teaching environment (Whitla et al., 2003); and thirdly that a demographically diverse medical school produces doctors with a greater awareness of the personal experiences of individuals from other socio-economic backgrounds (Grafton-Clarke et al., 2018).

The Foundation Year for Medicine at Edge Hill University has several features that support students' professional identity formation and active participation in medicine. These include:

- <u>Learning and Teaching is delivered in three-week blocks</u>. A focus is provided every three weeks to allow for meaningful connection to the content. For example, a topic might be 'children and young people' and delivered via 'real' world cases in small groups.
- <u>Assessments</u> are designed to not only reflect student progression and engagement but also support and mirror assessments in the coming years.
- <u>Two weeks of clinical shadowing experiences</u> in the community in recognition of the lack of opportunity for students to gain related experience (supports professional identity formation).
- <u>Induction week and transition days</u> and events to provide opportunities to discuss concerns with students in higher years of study (and peer mentoring).
- <u>Visit to regulatory bodies such as the General Medical Council (GMC)</u>. An opportunity to mix with other medical students and to speak to practicing doctors from diverse backgrounds.
- <u>Inter-professional learning days.</u> Students work through clinical cases with students on other professional training programmes (e.g., nurses and social workers).
- <u>Sessions on career pathways</u> provided by specialist careers advisors and medical practitioners.

- Clinical Skills and simulation days (not assessed but to support professional development).
- A Personal Academic Support tutor who supports students throughout medical training.
- Volunteering opportunities in the local community (e.g., Covid vaccination centres).
- Opportunities to engage with medical students nationally. This includes opportunities to join national committees and to attend funded national student conferences.
- Involvement (paid) in broader outreach initiatives that promote and broaden participation in medicine. This includes university outreach work to local colleges and summer schools. This supports evidence that found an increased acceptance of students who participated in outreach activities (Hammond et al., 2015).
- NHS Core skills and Public Health accreditation opportunities.
- Paid summer internships.
- Medical school societies (e.g., widening access to medicine society).
- Paid British Medical Association membership and free I-pad to support engagement and development of an electronic portfolio.
- Financial information and support. This includes financial advice sessions in the curriculum and the opportunity for students to apply for additional university grants (student support and hardship grants). This alleviates student's financial pressures and the need for widening participation students to take on paid work throughout training.

Initiatives to support students from widening access backgrounds during their undergraduate medical training

The National Medical School Widening Participation Forum has a Special Interest Group where staff from a wide variety of UK medical schools meet to share issues that they encounter in supporting medical students from widening access backgrounds and ideas and initiatives that have been implemented successfully in their institutions. Almost half of the medical schools in the UK are represented in this group, sharing good practice in supporting medical students from widening access backgrounds to participate more effectively in their medical education. Although improving financial support is key to enabling students from widening access backgrounds to make the most of opportunities whilst at medical school, the group has discussed many other initiatives that can have a positive impact on the experience and progression of these students. Some examples include:

- Practical ideas to minimise costs for students, for example, provision of 'scrubs'/clinical uniform, (University of Nottingham), provision of stethoscopes, facilitation of car-sharing for clinical placements, having rooms in the medical school open outside normal teaching times so students can study in the medical school and minimise fuel costs in rented accommodation, provision of food parcels.

- Provision of IT equipment (Edgehill University and University of Glasgow)
- Peer support with mentoring from more senior medical students (University of Manchester) www.bmh.manchester.ac.uk/study/medicine/apply/widening-access/
- Academic support – targeted for students who perform less well in formative assessments and individual, small group and online resources to help students develop their study and revision skills (University of Sheffield and Hull York Medical School) (Graham, 2023)
- Teaching about group work skills to embed a culture of inclusivity and help students learn effectively in problem-based learning groups (University of East Anglia)
- Using a patient's partnership group to help students prepare for clinical exams www.aru.ac.uk/health-medicine-and-social-care/medicine/patient-participation-group (Anglia Ruskin University)
- Mentoring by longitudinal one-on-one support from clinicians to raise aspirations, self-confidence, and belongingness by assisting professional socialisation, facilitating the development of a medical network, and supporting access to career development opportunities (University of Dundee)
- Personal tutor training to ensure personal tutors have an increased understanding of the needs of students from widening access backgrounds and senior tutor support (Aston University)
- Staff training, for example, reverse mentoring (Curtis et al., 2021)

In sharing experience of supporting medical students from diverse backgrounds, the group has discovered how different each medical school cohort can be. The proportion of medical students who live in their family home while studying varies significantly as does the proportion of medical students from minority ethnic groups. Such aspects can impact the support that medical students need to succeed, and consideration should be given to how appropriate support is best provided. For example, if students are commuting a long distance from their family home to the university rather than living in nearby student accommodation, it will be more difficult for them to participate in events outside normal working hours. There are important differences in financial provision for medical students across the four devolved nations in the UK, and variation in the selection criteria that are used to promote widening access with some giving greater priority to students from their own nation. Through discussion of students who face multiple challenges, for example, from social disadvantage, having English as a second language and having caring responsibilities for a family member, the impact of intersectionality has been highlighted. Each student will have had a unique journey to gaining a place at medical school and will have their own particular personal circumstances whilst they are studying medicine. It is important not to make assumptions about their needs and to value the diversity that students from widening access backgrounds bring to the medical school community.

Transition to working as doctors, postgraduate training, and future careers

Although medical students apply for their first jobs as doctors during the final year of their medicine course in the UK, in order to plan effectively for their future medical careers, they need to be thinking ahead from their early days at medical school. Those from widening access backgrounds may be satisfied with having successfully navigated the selection process for Medicine to be accepted onto their course and may not be looking ahead to their future medical career. Medical students who are, for example, the first in their family to go to university or who do not have a relative who is a doctor, may not be aware of the importance of building their curriculum vitae/personal portfolio while they are studying medicine. They may limit their vision to passing their assessments in order to graduate as a doctor and may not take advantage of opportunities that could help them in their future medical careers. Networking to build contacts while at medical school and seeking additional experiences such as audits, small research projects, academic presentations, and publications can enhance future postgraduate careers. Lack of awareness, finances, or time, for example, if students from widening access backgrounds are working in paid employment whilst being a student, can limit opportunities to take on additional roles and projects, attend events outside timetabled hours, or attend conferences. At some universities, it is possible for medical students to intercalate, that is, have a year out from their medical course in order to study for an additional degree. Medical students from widening access backgrounds may be less likely to consider intercalation because of the costs associated with an additional year of study (Nicholson et al., 2010). They may also lack the confidence or aspiration to consider studying for another degree while completing their primary medical qualification.

The application process for the UK Foundation Programme https:// foundationprogramme.nhs.uk/ to which most UK medical students will apply in order to start work as doctors has changed in recent years. Having prior degrees and publications are no longer credited in the application process for the 'standard' Foundation Programme. This revision of the application process can be viewed as having removed a level of disadvantage for students from widening access backgrounds who would be less able to afford the extra year's tuition fees and living costs usually needed to acquire an additional degree whilst at medical school.

A key change to the UK Foundation Programme application process that provides support for medical students from widening access backgrounds was introduced in 2022. Medical students who have entered their medicine course via a Widening Access Initiative, for example, Foundation/Gateway Year or via a contextual offer for a 'standard' medicine course and have been granted means-tested financial support whilst at medical school, can apply to work in the area of their medical school or the area of their home (usually family home). This initiative enables students from widening access backgrounds to have the social support of family and/or friends whilst starting their first jobs as doctors and living in the family home can potentially save them money on accommodation costs. Since this initiative was introduced, the majority of medical students at the University of Nottingham who have successfully completed the pre-allocation process have fulfilled the widening access criteria. This has made an important difference to many medical students as they embark on their first jobs after graduation.

The most recent change in the application process for the UK Foundation Programme has been to Preference Informed Allocation (2024 entry) following criticism of the fairness for minority groups of the previous system based on performance in medical school summative assessments or the national Situational Judgement Test exam (Sam et al., 2022). https://foundationprogramme.nhs.uk/programmes/2-year-foundation-programme/ukfp/

The current cohort of final-year students has yet to receive their Foundation Programme job allocation via this new process.

Application for the 'Specialised Foundation Programme', known formerly as the Academic Foundation Programme currently requires medical students to complete 'white space' questions to showcase their achievements beyond medical course assessments and credit is given for prior degrees, publications, and prizes awarded at medical school. These aspects of the application are normally used to shortlist for interviews. Medical students from widening access backgrounds are less likely to have chosen to intercalate and gain an additional degree and research opportunities while at medical school (Nicholson et al., 2010). They may lack the aspiration, confidence, or evidence to successfully apply to the Specialised Foundation Programme, thus missing an opportunity to gain research, leadership, management, or teaching experience as part of the UK Foundation Programme.

Case study – applying to the specialised foundation programme, Monisha Gupta, medical student who started in Foundation/Gateway Year, University of Nottingham

I found the Specialised Foundation Programme (SFP) application a frustrating and isolating experience. I have spent most of my free time during university working to earn money to fund the deficit caused by the NHS Bursary for my 5th and 6th years. I wasn't aware of the importance of getting publications or involvement in audits until it was close to the SFP application deadline, at which point it was too late. I felt disadvantaged compared to my counterparts, who had numerous audits and publications thanks to their connections with researchers and having more time and knowhow to complete them. I also couldn't access a lot of the resources to support SFP application due to their prohibitive costs.

During the final year of their medical training, students must also apply for provisional General Medical Council (GMC) registration, incurring additional expenditure. Following considerable pressure from groups such as the British Medical Association Students Committee, the GMC has recently announced that their registration fees for Foundation Year 1 doctors will be reduced.

Although there is awareness of the need to support students from widening access backgrounds through their undergraduate medical training, less consideration has been given to whether or not these students may continue to need support once they are doctors to enable them to successfully progress through postgraduate medical training. One example of a mentoring scheme for junior doctors from widening access backgrounds is 'RadReach' which provides mentors to support doctors who want to train to be radiologists www.rcr.ac.uk/career-development/professional-networks/radreach/the-radreach-mentoring-scheme/. Postgraduate medical exams are expensive, and doctors may enhance their chances of success by attending preparation courses that can also be costly. A recent report found that costs can vary between £330 and £1904, and may have a high failure rate, resulting in multiple resits, incurring further cost (Report Academy of Medical Royal Colleges, 2023) https://www.aomrc.org.uk/wp-content/uploads/2023/05/ATDG_Cost_of_postgraduate_training_0523.pdf. Completing postgraduate exams does not guarantee a future postgraduate training place.

Research has shown an association between having a widening access background and choice of career with students from a lower sociodemographic background being more likely to choose general practice as a career (Kumwenda et al., 2019). The relatively short postgraduate training to become a general practitioner in the UK and relatively high pass rate for the membership exam of the Royal College of General Practitioners www.rcgp.org.uk/mrcgp-exams alongside the competition ratios for other specialities may make general practice seem an attractive career option for students from widening access backgrounds. https://medical.hee.nhs.uk/medical-training-recruitment/medical-specialty-training/competition-ratios/2022-competition-ratios

In summary, university staff can help medical students to be better prepared for UK Foundation Programme application and later postgraduate medical training by providing good careers advice from the outset of an undergraduate medicine course. Financial support and encouragement for students who are academically able to successfully complete an intercalation year in order to gain an additional degree would also be valuable. In addition, providing learning opportunities to develop academic, management, and teaching skills will help all medical students to have a greater chance of success in applying for postgraduate training. Students from widening access backgrounds need individual support and guidance through the UK Foundation Programme application process if they wish to apply for pre-allocation to a particular area of the country, near either their medical school or their family home. For those who wish to apply for the Specialised Foundation Programme, support with completing application forms and interview preparation could help them succeed.

Future directions

In order for medical students from widening access backgrounds to not face the necessity of having paid employment during their medicine course, financial hardship needs to be addressed. During the later clinical years, either the NHS bursary should be increased, or universities need to continue to offer financial support. Providing more information to medical students from the outset of their undergraduate medical training about financial pressures during the later years of the course would enable them to plan ahead and, for example, work during longer vacations in the early years. Minimising hidden costs of undergraduate medical training will help all students especially those from widening access backgrounds. In the future, Medical Doctor degree apprenticeships will offer a new model of training in the UK, enabling future doctors to be paid whilst completing their undergraduate medical training. https://educationhub.blog.gov.uk/2023/06/30/nhs-doctor-apprenticeships-everything-you-need-to-know/

However, medical apprenticeships may prove to be controversial if aspiring medical students from widening access backgrounds are encouraged to pursue this route to qualification as doctors rather than the traditional university route, potentially creating a two-tiered system.

For students from widening access backgrounds on standard undergraduate medicine courses, having inspiring role models, either senior students or staff from diverse backgrounds, will encourage these medical students to feel they belong at medical school and therefore help them to succeed. Training for all staff working with medical students, to raise awareness of the increasing diversity of their social backgrounds should facilitate the provision of appropriate support and consideration of individual needs. Advice about careers especially application for postgraduate medical training, given from the outset of undergraduate medical course, would help students from widening access backgrounds to make the most of opportunities for building their personal portfolios whilst at medical school. Formalised career-building opportunities that are flexible around other commitments such as paid employment should be available to students from widening access backgrounds, to support personal portfolio and career development from the outset of their medical training. As medical students from widening access backgrounds graduate in increasing numbers, the institutions responsible for postgraduate medical training should consider the ongoing needs of these doctors. Greater provision of mentoring and a review of the costs associated with postgraduate medical exams will hopefully enable doctors from widening access backgrounds to progress into all specialities and enable a truly diverse medical workforce in the future.

References

Academy of Medical Royal Colleges. (2023). *The Cost of Medical Postgraduate Training Examinations: The Pressures, Challenges and Possible Remedies.* https://www.aomrc.org.uk/wp-content/uploads/2023/05/ATDG_Cost_of_postgraduate_training_0523.pdf

Anane, M., and Curtis, S. (2022). Is earning detrimental to learning? Experiences of medical students from traditional and low socioeconomic backgrounds. *British Student Doctor Journal*, 6(1), 14–22.

Berry, J., and Loke, G. (2011). Improving the degree attainment of Black and minority ethnic students. *Higher Education Academy and Equality Challenge Unit.* www.ecu.ac.uk/wp-content/uploads/external/improving-degree-attainment-bme

Cavanagh, A., Vanstone, M., and Ritz, S. (2019). Problems of problem-based learning: Towards transformative critical pedagogy in medical education. *Perspectives on Medical Education*, 8(1), 38–42.

Curtis, S., Mozley, H., Langford, C., Hartland, J., and Kelly, J. (2021). Challenging the deficit discourse in medical schools through reverse mentoring: Using discourse analysis to explore staff perceptions of underrepresented medical students. *BMJ Open*, 11(12), e054890. doi: 10.1136/bmjopen-2021-054890

Curtis, S., and Smith, D. (2020). A comparison of undergraduate outcomes for students from gateway courses and standard entry medicine courses. *BMC Medical Education*, 20, 1–14.

Dodsworth, E. (2024). *How Can We Improve Access to Healthcare Careers? How Can We Improve Access to Healthcare Careers?* universitiesuk.ac.uk

Foreshew, A., and Al-Jawad, M. (2022). An intersectional participatory action research approach to explore and address class elitism in medical education. *Medical Education*, 56(11), 1076–1085.

Grafton-Clarke, C., Biggs, L., and Garner, J. (2018). Why students from under-represented backgrounds do not apply to medical school. *Widening Participation and Lifelong Learning*, 20(1), 187–198.

Graham, A. (2023). https://asmepublications.onlinelibrary.wiley.com/doi/full/10.1111/tct.13657

Hammond, J., Dakin, C., White, H., Treadwell, E., and Grant, R. (2015). Ten years on: The long term impact of widening participation healthcare summer schools. *Widening Participation and Lifelong Learning*, 17(4), 49–66.

[HEE] Health Education England. (2014). *Widening Participation It Matters! Our Strategy and Initial Action Plan.* London: Health Education England.

Hmelo-Silver, C. E., and Barrows, H. S. (2006). Goals and strategies of a problem-based learning facilitator. *Interdisciplinary Journal of Problem-Based Learning*, 1(1), 4.

Krstić, C., Krstić, L., Tulloch, A., Agius, S., Warren, A., and Doody, G. A. (2021). The experience of widening participation students in undergraduate medical education in the UK: A qualitative systematic review. *Medical Teacher*, 43(9), 1044–1053. doi: 10.1080/0142159X.2021.1908976

Kumwenda, B., Cleland, J., Prescott, G., Walker, K., and Johnston, P. (2019). Relationship between sociodemographic factors and specialty destination of UK trainee doctors: A national cohort study. *BMJ Open*, 9(3), e026961. doi: 10.1136/bmjopen-2018-026961

Lave, J., and Wenger, E. (2001). Legitimate peripheral participation in communities of practice. *Supporting Lifelong Learning*, 1, 111–127.

Lok, P. (2022). *BMJ*, 377. doi: 10.1136/bmj.o1108 (accessed 3 May 2022)

Mann, K. V. (2011). Theoretical perspectives in medical education: Past experience and future possibilities. *Medical Education*, 45(1), 60–68.

McDuff, N., Hughes, A., Tatam, J., Morrow, E., and Ross, F. (2020). Improving equality of opportunity in higher education through the adoption of an inclusive curriculum framework. *Widening Participation and Lifelong Learning*, 22(2), 83–121.

Medical Schools Council. (2014). *Selecting for Excellence–Final Report*. www.medschools. ac.uk/media/1203/selecting-for-excellence-final-report.pdf

Medical Schools Council Selection Alliance Report. (2023). www.medschools.ac.uk/ news/selection-alliance-2023-report-published

Messiou, K. (2012). Collaborating with children in exploring marginalisation: An approach to inclusive education. *International Journal of Inclusive Education*, 16(12), 1311–1322.

Meuleman, A. M., Garrett, R., Wrench, A., and King, S. (2015). "Some people might say I'm thriving but . . . ": Non-traditional students' experiences of university. *International Journal of Inclusive Education*, 19(5), 503–517.

Mountford-Zimdars, A., Sabri, D., Moore, J., Sanders, J., Jones, S., and Higham, L. (2015). *Causes of Differences in Student Outcomes*. Report to HEFCE by King's College London, ARC Network and The University of Manchester. Bristol: HEFCE.

Munn, P., and Lloyd, G. (2005). Exclusion and excluded pupils. *British Educational Research Journal*, 31(2), 205–221.

Murray, A. (2022). www.bma.org.uk/news-and-opinion/medical-students-across-the-uk-are-feeling-the-financial-heat

Nemiroff, S., Blanco, I., Burton, W., Fishman, A., Joo, P., Meholli, M., and Karasz, A. (2023). Moral injury and the hidden curriculum in medical school: Comparing the experiences of students Underrepresented in Medicine (URMs) and non-URMs. *Advances in Health Sciences Education*, 1–17.

Nicholson, J. A., Cleland, J., Lemon, J., and Galley, H. F. (2010, March 23). Why medical students choose not to carry out an intercalated BSc: A questionnaire study. *BMC Medical Education*, 10(25). doi: 10.1186/1472-6920-10-25

Office for Students (OfS). (2019). *Access and Participation Plans*. [Online]. www. officeforstudents.org.uk/advice-andguidance/promoting-equal-opportunities/ access-and-participation-plans/

Reay, D., Crozier, G., and Clayton, J. (2010). "Fitting in"or "standing out": Working-class students in UK higher education. *British Educational Research Journal*, 36(1), 107–124.

Sam, A. H., Fung, C. Y., Reed, M., Hughes, E., and Meera, K. (2022). Time for preference-informed foundation allocation. *Clinical Medical Journal*, 11.

Sheeran, Y., Brown, B. J., and Baker, S. (2007). Conflicting philosophies of inclusion: The contestation of knowledge in widening participation. *London Review of Education*.

Singh, G. (2011). *Black and Minority Ethnic (BME) Students' Participation in Higher Education: Improving Retention and Success: A Synthesis of Research Evidence*. Heslington, UK: Higher Education Academy. https://www.advance-he.ac.uk/knowledge-hub/ black-and-minority-ethnic-bme-students-participation-higher-education-improving

Soria, K., and Bultmann, M. (2014). Supporting working-class students in higher education. *NACADA Journal*, 34(2), 51–62.

Whitla, D. K., Orfield, G., Silen, W., Teperow, C., Howard, C., and Reede, J. (2003). Educational benefits of diversity in medical school: A survey of students. *Academic Medicine*, 78(5), 460–466.

Yazdani, S., Andarvazh, M. R., and Afshar, L. (2020). What is hidden in hidden curriculum? A qualitative study in medicine. *Journal of Medical Ethics and History of Medicine*, 13.

Chapter 15

Drawing conclusions and future considerations

Louise Alldridge, Nana Sartania, Mandy Hampshire, Danielle Nimmons, Charlie Williams, Emily Róisín Reid, and Enam Haque

Introduction

When the idea for this book was first conceived, almost all UK medical schools had an agenda to widen participation. Although well-meaning their approaches were not rigorous or founded on a strong evidence base. Many activities were conflated with community engagement, and often lacked contemplation of pedagogy, efficacy, or intended learning outcomes. Similarly, there was a paucity of national evidence regarding inclusivity in medical selection processes. Consequently, groups of students outside of the perceived current 'norm' were unwittingly excluded from many medical schools and thus from a career in medicine.

In this book, we have shared experiences and best practices from members of the National Medical Schools Widening Participation Forum (NMSWPF) and hope these have proven to be both stimulating and informative for current and future practice. The Forum, and therefore this book, has brought together the views and expertise of a wide range of past and present practitioners, including Widening Participation Leads and Officers, students, practicing clinicians, and key members of organisations such as the Medical Schools Council. We have highlighted strategies currently or previously employed by medical schools across the student life cycle using case studies, research, evaluation, and discussions of best practice for building aspirations, engagement, selection, retention, success, and progression.

Drawing conclusions and future considerations

The book commenced by unpacking the meaning of widening participation and in its relevance in an elitist field. We recognised the unique setting of widening participation in medicine and began by demystifying and redefining it in a medical education setting. This sets the scene for all the proceeding chapters. Initially, we looked at novel, targeted outreach work across both primary and secondary schools. Many of the initiatives described incorporated informative practical guides which readers can adapt and utilise for outreach events across

DOI: 10.4324/9781003399858-15

diverse healthcare programmes. Other outreach activities integrated aspiration building with applied learning for school and beyond, including learning by engaging with cases, identifying strategies for effective independent study, application of new knowledge, and working alongside peers to solve problems. The activities, described in Chapter 2 not only improved communication skills for aspiring medical students but also enabled medical students, through designing and delivering the sessions, to develop their teaching skills and to engage with children from a wide range of age groups. In Chapter 3, we saw how embedding widening participation initiatives into the medical school curriculum (Student Selected Components), allowed fourth and later second-year medical students, to produce and deliver sustainable health educational and aspirational building material in local schools in deprived areas. The importance of engaging medical students in delivering and designing widening participation initiatives, regarding improving their appreciation of diversity and life chances as well as learning the art of teaching, is discussed further in Chapter 4.

As medicine encompasses several diverse careers, outreach activities can be adapted to help prospective students think about the wider range of careers in medicine. Chapter 5 details a unique and impactful initiative to not only increase the understanding of Psychiatry but to encourage pupils to consider it as a career along with a range of connected careers in Mental Health.

The book continues by exploring ways to enable WP students to complete their journey to becoming a doctor. Chapter 6 describes how targeted outreach interventions in Australia were followed up with transition initiatives and bespoke support. This led to successful graduation for students from Indigenous communities. The factors that were critical for their success can be and have been applied in WP strategies to medicine in the UK. This chapter highlighted how diversification of the medical profession had positive effects for the health of those they represent, illustrated by a significant increase in life expectancy for Indigenous people. Despite cultural difference, this work shows that having a medical profession that fully understands the people they treat has far-reaching consequences for the students' life chances but also health outcomes for the most under-represented groups.

The case studies shared in Chapter 7 illustrate that successful access work requires flexibility. The authors detail three different access programmes that are run in the same region of the north of England. Their differing structure, organisation, and approaches illustrate the diverse ways that aspiring medical students can successfully enter medical school.

Transitioning from a higher socio-economic background and a private school to medical school may be relatively easy for students equipped with social and cultural capital accrued from families and contacts matching that of the majority of students and educators. As we enrol more students from 'non-traditional' backgrounds, we need to ensure that the social and academic environment is inclusive and studying medicine is not an alienating experience for them. Chapter 8 discusses the social dynamics between the different groups. It provides the reader with some enlightening insights and outlines key strategies to help students from widening participation backgrounds to 'fit in' and thrive. This includes practical advice on recognising signs of isolation and initiatives to overcome this and develop a culture of support and acceptance.

Broadening out to a systemic focus, Chapter 9 reviews the progress and challenges, following the publication of the Medical Schools Council 'Selecting for Excellence Report', in 2014. This chapter looks at key initiatives, activities, and research conducted as well as the persisting challenges and future implications for widening participation in medicine.

In Chapter 10, we saw how it is possible to break down perceived barriers to medicine by providing realistic 'Champion' role models who helped young people from under-represented backgrounds to aspire to study medicine. Evaluation showed that both teachers and pupils were impressed by the role modelling by these champions. Three interventions to further enable smooth transition of WP students into medical school are outlined in Chapter 11. They cover supporting professional identity development but also practical workshops to enable students to tackle imposter syndrome and promote inclusivity.

Many medical schools use contextual markers to identify and verify WP applicants, however, many of these markers may not be precise and robust. As WP practitioners, we all want our students to come from a genuine WP background. Chapter 12 took a much-needed look at the system used to identify bonified WP candidates through evidence of backgrounds and personal circumstances. We all need to understand the efficacy of the data we use to determine whether a candidate is from a WP background and as illustrated in this book, we also need to know the implications of these markers and how each marker may link to potential support needs. In the future, these markers will not only be used for reduced entry requirements but also for targeted informed support as students move through their medical education and medical careers. As more WP students graduate and the tide moves further up the beach, there is growing recognition that processes for applying to UKFP allocation and selection for postgraduate training, and onward specialties, must change to ensure their selection systems are not classed and biased. For instance, there has been a move away from academic ranking for UK Foundation Programme (which involved points awarded for additional degrees and costly publications which are less accessible to WP students, particularly from Gateway Years) to a preference-informed, non-meritocratic allocation system with pre-allocation for WP students (UKFP, 2024). Recent changes have also been made in an attempt to make the Specialised Foundation Programme more accessible to those from WP backgrounds (UKFP, 2024).

Students from WP backgrounds generally thrive in medical school; however, their circumstances do not leave them, and many will need support as they progress through medical school. For these students, there is much to consider, and as time moves on more ways of supporting students and a clear focus on pedagogical considerations will emerge. Chapter 13 begins the quest to understand how educators and students from diverse backgrounds can interact in an educational setting to achieve best practice. Currently, teaching and learning practices remain embedded in classed and even gendered inequalities which influence how students and educators from different backgrounds engage in pedagogical spaces. Chapter 14 expands on some of the key issues faced by medical students from widening access backgrounds in medical school and the challenges encountered when they apply for their first jobs in the UK Foundation Programme and plan for future careers and postgraduate training application.

Most medical schools are proactively encouraging students from WP backgrounds by increasing the number of gateway programmes, rolling out of Medical Apprenticeships, and providing alternative contextual admissions routes. Therefore, it is imperative that all medical students receive appropriate and sufficient support. Staff should be acknowledging and understanding the impact of their students' background on their experiences at medical school and aim to accommodate them within the Medical School structures and processes. Institutions committed to widening participation should work hard to address and tackle underachievement on the course and beyond the medical school. This may be through designing new initiatives aimed at boosting students' self-esteem, involving students in voluntary work, and encouraging them to take part in competitions. Medical schools should all monitor the career destination of students from widening participation background and build strategies to level the postgraduate playing field. Above all, it will be essential to put in place central or local innovative ways to financially support these students.

Further future considerations should pay attention to detailed evaluation of new initiatives, such as medical school apprenticeships, to ensure parity of education and career trajectory with students graduating through the traditional route. Furthermore, attention should be paid to the large debt accrued, to ensure students from WP backgrounds are not affected at medical school or in future career choices. Initiatives such as mentoring for those from WP backgrounds from enrolment at medical school to consultant positions should be developed and implemented. We also need to acknowledge the intersectionality of students that we place in the bracket of WP. Understanding the diverse and unique struggles experienced by students categorised as 'WP' and putting in place bespoke solutions will be critical for success.

The future for pupils and medical students from under-represented demographics is definitely brighter than when the National Forum was formed. We have many more routes into medical careers, and there are opportunities to reduce financial hardship through the introduction of an Apprenticeship model of studying medicine. Selection procedures have and will continue to become more robust and ensure that students from WP backgrounds are selected through equitable processes. Our medical schools will develop their pedagogy to ensure it is inclusive and no longer a barrier to success for those from widening participation background. The impact of coming from a widening participation background will be understood, by all educators, and they will be supported appropriately during medical school, not only through inclusive pedagogy but equity in opportunities to help them reach their potential, leading to a truly representative medical workforce. As medicine and medical education diversify, there will be more equality of opportunity for all graduates and consequently a deeper understanding within the profession of the patients they treat. Finance remains a key barrier for these students, however, a report recently published by Universities UK (2024) concluded that one of the key ways to improve access to healthcare careers is to consider a student loan forgiveness scheme (UUK, 2024). This would be very welcome and transformative for students from widening participation backgrounds.

References

Foundation Programme (UKFP). (2024). https://foundationprogramme.nhs.uk/pro grammes/2-year-foundation-programme/ukfp/
How can we improve access to healthcare careers? Insights and Analysis, UUK. (2024). www.universitiesuk.ac.uk/latest/insights-and-analysis/how-can-we-improve-access-healthcare

Afterword

Our aim in writing this book was to share and reflect on the changes and insights brought about through the work of the National Widening Participation Forum, whose vision is to promote best practice in widening participation in UK medical schools and to act as a problem-solving and supportive forum for widening participation leads in Medicine. The Forum revived and energised Widening Participation in medical schools, whose work was often conflated with marketing and community engagement. Prior to the work of the Forum and the Medical Schools Council, little thought was given to pedagogy, in-depth analysis of the efficacy, and ultimate outcomes of widening participation interventions. Similarly, selection processes employed often disenfranchised certain groups or individuals, thus exacerbating under-representation.

We have explored different pedagogical approaches employed by medical schools to help under-represented students to access medicine, transition smoothly to and thrive in the medical school environment, and beyond. We hope this book can act as a practical guide for widening participation in medicine and other 'elite' programmes and careers. The contents are based on proven efficacy, practitioner expertise, evaluation, and research. As many barriers still exist, and we hope that some of the studies recounted in this book will not only inform but trigger further research and investigations as widening participation continues to change and evolve. As we increase the number of students from Widening Access backgrounds, our medical schools will need to look closely at the traditional pedagogies that still underpin much of our teaching, learning, and assessment. In making evidence-based and sometimes radical changes, we can ensure our target groups are not impeded from succeeding in medical school and progressing to their careers of choice but can flourish.

We anticipate that this book will also have a broader impact, as medical education policy and practice can be generalised across many countries. Although the work is mostly UK-based, the content is relevant and transferrable. Efforts to increase social justice in medical education is a feature in other countries, particularly Canada, Germany, and Australia, as noted in the work to widen participation of Indigenous, first nation people in an Australian medical school.

Looking through a wider lens, the future of our healthcare system and our own health is in many ways determined by the Doctors that we select and educate. In a diverse country, it is vital that we have a healthcare workforce that understands not only the conditions they treat but the breadth of the social and psychological narratives of their patients. As such, together we are making progress towards the BMA's statement in 2009, that 'Doctors should be as representative as possible of the society they serve in order to provide the best possible care to the UK population.'

Index